The Cutting Edge

Reflections & Memories by Doctors on Medical Advances in Reno

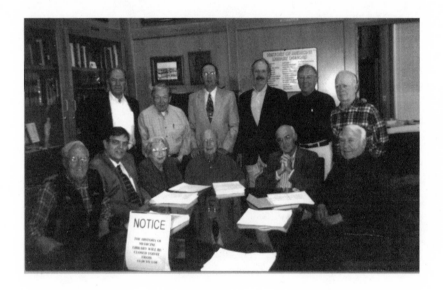

Titles in the Golden Age of Medicine in Nevada Series

The Cutting Edge

Reflections & Memories by Doctors on Medical Advances in Reno

Richard G. Pugh   Greasewood Press Ⓨ Reno

G R E A S E W O O D   P R E S S
PATHOLOGY/350 RENO, NEVADA 89557

Manufactured in the United States of America

Book design by Anton Sohn
Book formatting by Teresa Garrison
Dust Jacket photography by William J. Thompson

FIRST   PRINTING

1 2 3 4 5 6 7 8 9

Production of *The Cutting Edge* was made possible
By grants from The John Ben Snow foundation,
The School Medicine's Department of Pathology,
and the Nevada History of Medicine Foundation

Library of Congress Catalog Card Number and
CIP data are located at end of book

Contents

Illustrations

Abbreviations, Definitions, and Acronyms

5-FU	5-Fluorouracil
ACL	Anterior cruciate ligament
AD	Alzheimer's disease
AIDS	Acquired Immunodeficiency Syndrome
AMA	American Medical Association
ANGIOGRAPHY	The study of blood vessels by using radio-opaque dyes
ANGIOPLASTY	Surgical repair of blood vessels
BIRD	Respirator invented by Forrest M. Bird
BPH	Benign prostatic hypertrophy
CABG	Coronary artery bypass graft
CAT SCANNER	Computed axial tomography scanner (also CT scanner)
CCC	Civilian Community Corps for work on public land
CHAMPUS	Civilian Health & Medical Program of the Uniformed Services
CNS	Central nervous system
CPAP	Continuous positive airway pressure
CPM MACHINE	Continuous passive motion machine
CULPOSCOPE	Equipment for examination of the cervix
CYTOGENETICS	Study of cells that contain genetic material
CYTOLOGY	Study of cells to determine malignancy
DNA	Deoxyribonucleic acid (genetic material in the cell)
DRG	Diagnostic Related Groups
DTS	Delirium tremens
ECHOCARDIOGRAM	Sonogram of the heart
ECT	Electro-convulsive therapy
ED	Erectile dysfunction
EKG	Electrocardiograph (tracing of the heart's electrical beat)
ESTERASE	Enzyme found in white blood cells
ENDOSCOPE	A tube that is inserted into body
FACTOR VIII	Protein necessary for blood coagulation
FDA	Food and Drug Administration
FIBEROPTIC	Visualization under the skin through a small tube
GENOME	Set of chromosomes in the cell
GI	Gastrointestinal

GI	Government-issue
GP	General Practitioner
HAWC	Health Access in Washoe County
HEMATOLOGY	Study of blood disorders
HEMOCYTOMETER	A glass chamber where blood cells are counted visually
HEPATITIS	Viral infection of the liver
HMO	Health Maintenance Organization
HPV	Human Papilloma Virus
HRPC	Hormonal resistant prostate cancer
IMMUNOLOGY	Study of immunity
IN UTERO	Formed inside the uterus
IN VITRO	Formed outside of the body
IV	Intravenous
IVP	Intravenous pyelorgram
LAPAROSCOPE	A small tube that is inserted into the abdomen
LASIK	Laser-assisted keratotomy
LAUP	A surgical laser procedure to remove uvula
LEEP	Loop electrocautery excision procedure for biopsies
LITHOTRIPTER	A device that employs ultrasound to pulverize stones in body
LMC	Laboratory Medicine Consultants
MCAT	Medical College Admission Test
MRI	Magnetic resonance imaging (visualizes anatomy)
NIAAA	National Institute on Alcoholism and Alcohol Abuse
NIDA	National Institute of Drug Abuse
NIH	National Institute of Health
NSAIDS	Nonsteroidal anti-inflammatory drugs
NSMA	Nevada State Medical Association
OTC	Over the counter
PCR	Polymerase chain reaction (test that amplifies DNA)
PERINATOLOGY	Specialty focusing on the birth period
PET	Positron emission tomography (visualizes injected isotopes)
PMMA	Polymethylmethacrylate
PPO	Preferred Provider Organization
PSA	Prostatic specific antigen (protein in prostate tissue)
PSP	Prostatic acid phosphatase (enzyme in prostate tissue)
PSRO	Professional Standards Review Organization
RK	Radial keratotomy
SAMI	State Aid to the Medically Indigents

SEROLOGY	Study of proteins in the serum
SMH	Saint Mary's Hospital
SNL	Sierra Nevada Laboratories
SONOGRAM	Use of sound waves to identify anatomy
TOXICOLOGY	Study of drugs and foreign chemicals in the body
TURP	Transurethral Resections of Prostate
UNSOM	University of Nevada School of Medicine
URINALYSIS	Analysis of urine
WASHOE	Washoe Medical Center
WBC	White blood cell
WHS	Washoe Health System
WMC	Washoe Medical Center

Acknowledgments

Researching the advances in medicine for this book was an adventure and a learning experience. I had the honor and pleasure of working with many fine, dedicated physicians, but most of the credit goes to Drs. Frank Roberts, John Davis, Rodney Sage, Anton Sohn, and Owen Bolstad, who initiated the idea behind this book. From them and the other doctors who provided the material in this book, I received a "crash course" in medicine as it has been practiced in northern Nevada over the last five decades. These doctors provided the enthusiasm for *The Cutting Edge*, and it was a sad day when Dr. Bolstad passed away half way through the process.

Linda Fine was the original researcher and interviewer for this book and deserves credit for organizing and setting the stage for the interviews that followed. She had to retire due to her husband's illness, but her touch is present throughout the book.

The clerical and administrative staff of the History of Medicine Program and Pathology Department in the University of Nevada School of Medicine did a major part of this work. They kept the mood light while getting everything done on schedule. I had the pleasure of working with Gussie Burgoyne, Linda McLellan, and Teresa Garrison. I certainly want to acknowledge the encouragement and support of friend, publisher, and editor, Anton Sohn, M.D., whose sense of the importance of medical history in Nevada kept us on track.

The medical specialists selected for chapters in this book gave their time and insights graciously, and none held back on their opinions and oftentimes-sensitive issues. Each has made a substantial contribution to medicine, and their collective wisdom will always be a part of the medical culture in northern Nevada.

Foreword

With the advancement of knowledge in all fields of science, particularly in medicine, longevity and quality of life have dramatically increased during the last fifty years. The standard of medical care has continued to extend life expectancy from under fifty years to seventy-five years and beyond; patients in northern Nevada have benefited from this change. The Silver State has experienced this medical advancement as doctors trained elsewhere have chosen this state as a quality place to live and practice their art. They brought new knowledge, thus helping to deliver the state-of-the-art medical care we enjoy. By moving to northern Nevada these physicians fulfilled their dreams and shared their knowledge with colleagues to help deliver a high standard of medical care.

In the early days of Nevada medicine, the low demand for services of many medical specialties created the necessity to send some patients to areas where they could obtain more advanced care. In the last forty years, with the population growing and with the development of the University of Nevada School of Medicine, demand grew for local specialty services and new, well-trained specialists were attracted to northern Nevada. Today, except in extremely unusual circumstances, the necessity for a patient to go out of state for care is rare. In fact, the contrary is true as patients from other states frequently travel here for medical care.

The accomplishments of the medical community in promoting high standards of care in northern Nevada have come about, for the most part, through the efforts of physicians, hospitals, medical societies, and local, state, and federal governments. As a result of this cooperation, much has been done, but there are many issues, such as the shortage of physicians in rural areas and lack of affordable health insurance for everyone, left to be resolved in the future.

This book covers the advances in medicine as seen through the eyes of over a dozen specialty and sub-specialty physicians who settled here and made the medical community what it is today—a truly state-of-the-art medical center.

John Iliescu, M.D.

The Cutting Edge

Reflections and Memories by Doctors on Medical Advances in Reno

1: Introduction

A Brief Look at the History of Medicine

There is nothing more dynamic or that affects more lives worldwide than the progress of medicine. The field of medicine is constantly changing through advances in science and technology, ethical values, delivery systems, and the use of non-M.D. practitioners, just to name a few. As a result, the role of the team captain—the physician, is also changing. Physicians have not been passive observers of the miracles and wonders occurring over the last half of the twentieth century. In fact, they have been the catalysts that have brought about most of these life-extending and life-improving miracles. Unfortunately, in the last fifty years, the art of medicine has been moved aside somewhat by science and technology. Although the art and humanity of medicine are still important, our society is placing more emphasis on technological advances, which have resulted in increased specialization. A trained physician cannot possibly know how to use all the high tech instrumentation used within his or her specialty and this has led to the creation of differing levels of medical-technological assistants.

In 1950 five years after the United States successfully concluded the war against Japan and Germany, the population of Nevada was 160,000 scattered over 110,540 square miles, but that represented a forty-five percent increase over the 1940 census. Nevada was growing. Even though Las Vegas was barely a crossroads, the northern part of the Silver State represented just about everything that was considered Nevada, namely, gaming and divorce. Reno and its neighbor, Sparks, were tiny river towns situated between Salt Lake City and San Francisco on two-lane U.S. Highway 40 and the Southern Pacific railroad. What medical technology that had filtered into the state was primarily located in Reno. By 1940 technological advances had slowly entered the state, but opportunities for the latest in cutting-edge patient care would be obtained principally by traveling to other areas, such as San Francisco, Salt Lake City, or even back East.

In those early days physicians carried most of their scientific wonders in their black leather bags and, during the era of house calls, were able to carry most of what modern medicine could offer in that small bag. Penicillin for infections, laudanum for pain, and palliative medications were there for persistent chronic diseases and stubborn health conditions. They were aware of aseptic techniques for fighting infections and used vaccinations routinely. Nevada doctors, working through their scientific organizations such as the Nevada State Medical Association and the AMA, showed a keen interest in solving public health problems like polio, measles, smallpox, tuberculosis, and respiratory illness prevalent in the hard rock mining industry. Specialty societies were formed and assumed the role of educators by keeping their members informed of medical advances.

Advances in the science and practice of medicine were sporadic over the past three thousand years because most innovative thinkers who challenged the accepted theories of disease were ridiculed and most of the time ostracized by their contemporaries. In order to understand the advances in medical practice in Reno that have transpired during the past fifty years, it would be wise to briefly consider the great thinkers and physicians who have influenced the medical profession since the beginning of western civilization.[1]

In the western world, prior to the ancient Greeks, disease was considered the province of the supernatural and the solely the result of a displeased Supreme Being. (One can't help but reflect on how some religious groups explained the recent AIDS epidemic.) In the sixth century B.C., Greek philosophers began to look at disease as a natural phenomenon and believe sickness was due to an imbalance of natural powers within the body. Hippocrates (460-379 B.C.), who is the "Father of Medicine," defined these as black bile, yellow bile, phlegm (mucus), and blood.

Shortly after Hippocrates' death, the control of the western world shifted to Rome, but the Greeks still led the way in medical thinking. Their next great physician was Galen (159-203 A.D.) whose fame spread to Rome where he moved to serve as physician to the emperor. Galen made numerous anatomical discoveries and attributed disease to organ dysfunction, but he persisted in believing the existence of Hippocrates' four humors. His ideas lasted through the Middle Ages, but challenges began to occur in the Renaissance. Leonado da Vinci (1452-1519) made brilliant drawings of human anatomy, and Andreas Versalius further stimulated the field of anatomy through his sketches and descriptions of the cadaver. Another contemporary of da Vinci's was the physician, Paracelsus, who advanced the idea of empirical treatment of disease and introduced mercury for the treatment of syphilis and the use of laudanum (an alcoholic solution of opium) for pain.

The pace quickened in the seventeenth century and important advances moved the practice of medicine forward. The seventeenth century was an age of discovery and maybe its greatest physician was William Harvey (1578-1657). In his great monogram, *de Motu Cordis* he demonstrated that blood actually circulated throughout the body. Fifty years later, Anton Van Leewenhoek (1632-1723) studied "little animals" under his microscope. Then an explosion of discoveries occurred: smallpox vaccination-1796, anesthesia-1848, x-rays-1895, electrocardiograms (EKG)-1902, and eventually the discovery of DNA and its vast implications for advances in genetics came later in the twentieth century.

Just two hundred years ago many physicians held to the ancient belief there were four humors—mucus, blood, black bile, and yellow bile, that, when in harmony and balance, resulted in good health. Bloodletting, which restored this balance, became one of the physician's primary weapons against illness and a badge of his profession. Another philosophy, dating back to the time of Plato, held that symptoms could be grouped into entities defining specific diseases.

Scarcely sixty years before World War II the bacterial cause of disease was discovered, and the war years introduced the "golden bullet"—antibiotics—which resulted in a marked increase in the quality of life.

New medical science and technology added to the growing library of knowledge composing "modern medicine" in the United States, but none of the great scientific advances originated in northern Nevada. In fact, these discoveries might have arrived in the Silver State a long time—decades even, after being introduced in the great research centers of the world. Yet, doctors in the Silver State were proud, even boastful, of their status as being "state of the art" in providing medical care day in and out in this sparsely populated state. At the 1915 meeting of the Nevada State Medical Society (now the Nevada State Medical Association), after hearing a scientific paper on the x-ray as a valuable "aid" in setting a fracture, a doctor commented, "Any doctor who cannot set a broken bone without the use of x-ray should have his license revoked!" After all, Nevada's doctors lived on the frontier and survived by their wits and skills when technology was not available.

As late as 1962, interns on the wards of San Francisco General Hospital, which was under the auspices of University of California and Stanford medical school, were doing blood counts using a hemocytometer invented by Sir Richard Gowers in 1877. Blood electrolytes, a test considered today to be indispensable for twenty-four hour critical patient care, was only available during the forty-hour work week and the clinical laboratory and the radiology laboratory were relegated to out-of-the-way spaces in the basements of most hospitals.

Today, high technology equipment, such as the computed axial tomography scanners (CAT), the magnetic resonance imaging scanners (MRI), and the positron emission tomography scanners (PET) are all located prominently and are the showcase of today's modern hospital.

During the period covered in this book, physician's offices were beginning to enjoy modernity also. There were advances in office technology and the doctor's outer office benefited through the use of electronics, such as typewriters, fax machines, automated billing systems, dictation equipment, telephone systems, and later specialized computer systems.

By the 1960s, the art and science of medicine in Nevada began a steady rise to what it is today—"state of the art' in every respect. Only in very rare instances today is a patient referred out of state for treatment and in many of those cases such referral is necessitated by the rarity of the disease or the patient's desire to get an outside opinion.

It is becoming increasingly evident that delivery of quality medical care is becoming quite expensive, both to the providers of that care and those receiving it. Could it be the steady increase in healthcare and medical costs, (never mind the awesome benefits of these medical-technological advances) has caused thousands of Nevadans and millions of American to seek what is commonly called "alternative" healthcare with its "natural" remedies, potions, elixirs, and modalities? In the face of such monumental technological advances that have swept the land over the last half of the twentieth century, it is a curious thing that so many people are opting to try experimental, unproven, and potentially dangerous healthcare "alternatives." In defense of modern medical technology, however, even a casual observer would see that men and women from all over the world come to these shores to avail themselves of our advanced medical care; they do not come for "alternative" and unproven remedies and treatments.

That casual observer would find it extremely interesting, too, were he to look back on the legislative adventures of the Nevada State Medical Association over the past three decades to see that Nevada lawmakers began taking a serious look at the expense of healthcare and took it upon themselves to change directions of that system in non-scientific ways.

In the 1971 session, a bill was introduced to authorize the addition of a new system of health and medical care called "acupuncture." Lobbyists said passage of the bill would be the answer to the rising costs of health care in the Silver State and $5 healthcare treatments would become a reality once again. Robert Broadbent, M.D., a Reno general practitioner elected to the legislature in 1970, began an extensive lobbying effort early in the 1971 session to inform his Assembly colleagues of the pitfalls of licensing people with dubious credentials to practice a form of medicine of little or no proven scientific value. He cautioned them to be wary of outrageous testimonials and anecdotal revelations and tried, to no avail, to build support for defeat of the bill or, as a back up position, to set up an interim study of the matter. However, Governor Mike O'Callaghan signed the bill licensing the practice of acupuncture in the state, ignoring the objections and petitions of the state's 1,000 medical doctors. Assemblyman Broadbent, disillusioned with the whole legislative process, did not offer for re-election.

There are few acupuncturists practicing in Nevada today, and it is worth noting that once acupuncture was licensed in 1971, $5 office visits never materialized. This form of alternative treatment never had a measurable effect on either reducing health care costs or improving patient outcomes in Nevada. It is evident that acupuncture did not meet the test of public acceptance then and it is not widely accepted today.

Another example of legislative maneuvering into the healthcare arena, ostensibly to contain healthcare costs, was the passage of a bill in 1977 authorizing the manufacture, sale, and use of the alleged cancer-curing substance called Laetrile. The passage of a health and vitality enhancing elixir called Gerovital was equally ineffective. These unproven, expensive substances did not enrich the lives of those who used them, but they certainly enriched the coffers of lobbyists and manufactures who pushed these measures through the legislature.

In legislative sessions in the late 1970s and early 1980s lobbyists for commercial interests were working overtime for passage of a law establishing the practice of "naturopathy" in Nevada. Lobbyists said that a naturopath was a person with special skills and training, who treats a host of maladies in a very inexpensive and natural way. In previous legislative sessions medical lobbyists defeated naturopathy legislation by pointing out that it had no demonstrable value and was potentially dangerous to the health of Nevadans. The protection of the health of the public has always been a basic tenet of the medical profession. It came as a surprise when the naturopathic bill was passed in 1981 over the objection of physicians, who were consumed with passage of major tort reform legislation. The practice of naturopathy in Nevada proved to be an embarrassment to the legislature for the next several years and was eliminated from the statutes in 1985.

In the 2002 book, *Serving Medicine*, Larry Matheis, executive director of the Nevada State Medical Association, commented, "The healthcare system now involves many players other than physicians." One of the players is the state legislature, but the principal players are people who are willing to experiment with their health even if that experimentation can be proven not to be in their best interest. The wish for "freedom of choice" in healthcare goes hand-in-hand with a fascination of the unproven treatment, and it competes with all the wonderful advances in procedures, drugs, and medical technology.

Medical technology in the United States will continue its advances whether or not the entire population fully appreciates or accepts its benefits. The costs will be borne by patients, governmental entities, and investors. It is conceivable that the next modern medical technological advances with life saving and increasing longevity potential will be a financial threat to the U.S. healthcare system.

Recently we observed Vice President Richard Cheney have a state-of-the-art defibrillator implanted in his chest. This devise can detect an abnormal heart rhythm and supply a small electrical current to bring the heart rate back to normal rhythm, thereby preventing a cardiac death. The dilemma is that the devise costs over $20,000 and operation to implant it costs another $10,000. A recent study by Dr. Arthur Moss in the *New England Journal of Medicine* reported that as many as four million Americans have a cardiac condition similar to Cheney's, and as many as 400,000 new patients a year may need this defibrillator.[2] Moss estimated that seventy percent of those four million are covered under the Medicare program. Simple math indicates this could create an expense for the program of $84 billion for this one procedure. The entire Medicare budget this year is approximately $220 billion and approving this procedure could bankrupt this valuable program and destroy private insurers within a short period of time.

Not to be forgotten, in the ever-increasing costs of medical care, are those expenses created by physicians who are forced to practice defensive medicine. It is a certainty that somewhere in early medical-legal literature is documentation of a suit against a hospital or physician for needing, but not having available, a CAT scanner, or an MRI, or some other high tech piece of equipment. The threat of a malpractice suit inevitably creates the need for the very latest in medical technology, which directly leads to increased healthcare costs.

In this book we interview numerous physicians in medical specialties who have practiced in northern Nevada since the 1950s. In their words, doctors will outline reasons why they chose northern Nevada to practice and raise their families, and how they perceived the medical community when they arrived. We will explore first-hand the important technological and scientific advances that evolved in their specialty and will examine how these advances changed their practice and benefited their patients.

Notes

[1] For a more complete history of medicine see Ackerknecht's *A Short History of Medicine*.

[2] Moss, Arthur, et al, "Prophylactic Implantation of a Defibrillator in Patients with Myocardial Infarction and Reduced Ejection Fraction" *NEJM,* March 21, 2002, Vol. 346, No. 12, pp. 877-83.

2: Dr. Ronald Cudek, Anesthesia

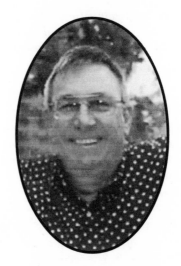

Dr. Ronald Cudek

Education

I was born April 8, 1935, in East Chicago, Indiana, and raised in Whiting, Indiana, in an area known as "The Region." We lived right on the state line between Gary and Chicago. I earned an undergraduate degree from Wabash College, which is in Crawfordsville, Indiana. It is one of the top small liberal arts schools in the country.

My mother was responsible for my going into medicine. Ever since I was a little kid, she was always saying, "Be a doctor or dentist and be your own boss," and that proved to be good advice, but that prodding from my mother also caused me to rebel somewhat. Maybe, I thought, since it wasn't really my idea, it might be something I didn't want to do.

At Wabash I took classes that would have led to a degree in chemistry, with a minor in math, until my advisor informed me in my junior year, "You haven't taken any classes in zoology or biology even though you signed up for premed." He said. "I think you ought to have at least a second minor in zoology." So that's what I did. I realized there was not much of a future in chemistry so I started taking lots of courses in zoology and biology, and in my senior year I took the medical school aptitude test. Even then, I wasn't completely sold on the medical school idea and felt I was taking the test for my mom. I passed and applied at Northwestern University and Indiana University medical schools. As my family was by no means wealthy, it would have been a strain on their finances if I went to Northwestern, so, when Indiana, our state-supported school, accepted me during the interview, I accepted their offer by enrolling in

1957 and graduating in 1961.

There was still some reluctance to pursue a medical career until I actually got into the classes, then it was like turning on a light. One day in an anatomy lab I remember saying to myself, "Hey! This is for me. Yeah, I think this is going to be all right." Going into medicine and becoming a doctor, however, was not a life long dream coming true.

After medical school, I knew I wanted to go West for my internship. I didn't know where exactly in the West I would go, but during medical school, I did externships in San Francisco and at a mental hospital in Sedro Woolley, Washington. I particularly liked Washington; I applied and was accepted for an internship in Tacoma and moved there in 1961.

Internship and Residency

During my general internship, we did everything. Emergency room medicine wasn't a specialty yet, and for a six-week period, I was the only emergency room physician at the hospital. I did obstetrics for six weeks and delivered a lot of babies at that county hospital. Next were six-week rotations in pediatrics, medicine, and surgery. It was a very well rounded internship—made more well rounded by the fact that Phyllis and I got married. I had met her in my senior year at med school and we were married in 1962.

I did meet a lot of super people there and I remember one man, in particular, who interested me in specializing in anesthesia: Dr. John Bonica, head of the department. He was well known for his work in pain blocking with regional anesthesia and had built quite a reputation throughout the world. John worked his way through med school as a professional wrestler and became famous as "The Masked Marvel." The University of Washington enticed him to become head of its anesthesia department in Seattle, which he accepted on the condition that it included his Tacoma anesthesia program.

I got to know a lot of the anesthesia residents there and just fell into that specialty because my colleagues strongly encouraged me to consider it. Actually, I was considering ophthalmology, but I liked the applied physiology involved in anesthesiology, as physiology was my favorite subject in medical school. Another plus was that if I entered an anesthesia residency, I could stay in Tacoma where I already had a lot of friends and wouldn't have to move again. I was ready to settle down.

I finished my two-year residency program at Tacoma in 1962 and for a three-month period, commuted to Seattle for my training in cardiovascular anesthesia, which was just beginning in those days. I can remember every morning getting up about four o'clock to drive up to

Seattle. There were no freeways at that time, and we had to drive right past the Boeing plant to get to Seattle. Mornings weren't that bad because it was early enough that I didn't hit much traffic, but if I got done early in the afternoon and had to come back at four or five o'clock. Boeing traffic was just awful. Overall my wife, Phyllis, and I enjoyed our stay in Tacoma and two of our sons, Scott and Adam, were born there.

U.S. Navy

I finished my residency in 1964 and entered the service. In 1957, before entering med school, I had my draft physical examination, and the doctor asked me if I had ever had trouble with my knee. I told him it was a football injury. After the exam I was tagged "4-F." Shortly after graduating from medical school, I received a draft notice addressed to "Dr. Cudek," and that was a tip-off they knew I was a doctor. I informed them that I had been rated "4-F," and they quickly informed me that I was alive, breathing, and had a pulse, so I was officially in the draft. Evidently my 4-F status counted only as a deferment and my becoming a doctor put a whole new light on my eligibility. I was offered the Berry Plan as an alternative, allowing me to finish my residency training. I was enlisted in the navy, but never went to meetings or anything for the next two years. Just before completing my training, the navy asked where I would like to be stationed. I gave them quite a variety of places that interested me: Bremerton, Washington; San Diego, California; and Washington, DC. Where did they send me? Key West, Florida!

We traveled across the country in a VW bug, camping out all the way. Phyllis and the boys slept in the car and I slept outside, occasionally under the car when it rained. I was a lot thinner at that time. That little car, even the roof rack, was loaded to the max.

When I reported to the commanding officer at the Key West Naval Hospital, I said, "Hi, I'm Dr. Cudek, I'm your new anesthesiologist." The captain looked at me and growled, "Where's your uniform?" I told him I never had one. Then he asked about my basic training and I told him I didn't get any. There was another officer in the corner of the commander's office about to split a gut laughing who was told, "Lt. Mousel, take this man and get him a uniform." That officer turned out to be Dr. Donald Mousel who would later move to Reno to practice ophthalmology.

Don took me to the commissary where I was outfitted with a uniform. We then returned to the commanding officer, who shouted, "Where's your hat? You're out of uniform." "They're on back order. They didn't have any in stock," I replied. You would have thought I was a traitor. Lt. Mousel was cracking up again, and I couldn't keep a straight face either. The captain loaned me one of his hats to wear.

I became chief of anesthesia at the Key West Naval Hospital. It was a grand title, but I was the only anesthesiologist on the base. There was one nurse anesthetist, and we shared call every other night, but fortunately we weren't that busy. She happened to get pregnant and was discharged out of the service, leaving me for about three months by myself, with twenty-four hour call, seven days a week, 365 days, but it really wasn't all that bad.

Move to Reno

Dr. Don Mousel and I worked together for a year and we became best friends before he completed his military service that year. He moved to Reno and kept me informed of goings-on there, and I began to take an interest in relocating to Reno when my hitch was up. I asked him to check to see if there were any openings for anesthesiologists; he found out there was an opening, so I flew to Reno to check it out. It was a little tough getting to Reno as I was flying military standby. The military thought I was trying to book a flight to "Rio."

When I got to town, I stayed with the Mousels and interviewed for the position. Don showed me around and took me on a tour of everything in the area. We went out to Pyramid Lake and were entertained by a couple of Native Americans playing guitars in one of the bars there and had a super time. Later, we flew over to Winnemucca in a private plane arranged by one of Don's friends, a judge named Jack Matthews, and while there, another of Don's friends, a local dentist, gave us a tour of the red light district. We actually went into one of the houses, the Cozy Corner. It was being remodeled at the time and the madam showed us around, but we did no business there. After that tour, I thought, "Hey! This is a pretty interesting part of the country."

When I got back to Key West, I told Phyllis we were heading to Reno and she readily agreed to it. Our third son, Todd, was born in Key West, and she was expecting our fourth, Aaron, who would be born in Reno. So the "five and a half" of us drove back to Reno in the dead of summer, but this time we had a van (no air conditioning) and towed the Volkswagen Bug.

Anesthesia in Reno

Reno Anesthesiologists

Anesthesia in Reno was state of the art in every respect. I checked that out with Dr. John Bonica in Washington when I was considering moving here. The anesthesia community in Reno consisted of Drs. Bob Crosby, Arthur Scott, Bill O'Brien, Dave Williams, Jack Flanary, and Bill Simpson.[1]

Drs. Dick Kaiser and Barney Barnstein would join us a year or so later. Dr. Charles McCuskey, Sr., was also working part-time. Dr. Bonica commented that the practice in Reno was the best private practice in the United States at the time. I found the technology, techniques, and the quality of anesthesia to be of the highest level. And surprisingly, there were no nurse anesthetists in the area. I think when some of the first anesthesia M.D.s came to town, there were nurses in the field, but, as more and more physicians came, that practice stopped.

Reno had a well-organized medical community and I was asked from time to time to get involved in medical politics, but almost always declined. St. Mary's administration approached me to head up the pharmacy committee one year and I agreed to do that as long as it didn't lead to any other political jobs. I later was asked to consider being chief of staff at St. Mary's, but I asked, "Why would I want to be that?" In response to that question I got, "Being chief of staff would be a great honor." I said, "I don't want to be chief of staff," and turned it down. They never asked me again.

When I did my training back in the early 1960s with Dr. Bonica, Tacoma was the nerve block center of the world. In fact, that's how he became world famous because he was a big advocate of regional anesthesia and wrote a textbook on it. In my training under him we did most things under a local block. We did thyroid surgery under cervical blocks and abdominal surgeries under epidural anesthesia. At the time this was not being done around the country. In obstetrics, I would guess that over ninety-five percent of the deliveries there were done under caudal epidural anesthesia. In fact, it became "funny" because women really didn't care who their obstetrician was as long as they had a caudal anesthesia. I had a lot of regional anesthesia training and brought that training and technology with me to Reno. Patients loved it and doctors loved it too; patients were nice and comfortable, it was a very safe procedure, and deliveries were speeded up.

Advances in Anesthesiology

There have been a lot of advances in the practice of anesthesia over the years, and I think this has prompted advances in other surgical specialties. New drugs have come along and the technology of anesthesia has also advanced. As a resident administering anesthesia to a senior citizen, say, a seventy-plus year old patient, it was always a challenge. Toward the end of my practice, it was not uncommon to administer anesthesia, on an outpatient basis, to one-hundred-year old patients.

My colleagues joke about anesthesia, saying things like, "Putting patients to sleep is the easy part—bringing them out is the hard part," and I frequently have been quoted as telling my patients, "I don't charge you anything for putting you to sleep—all I charge for is waking you up."

In the 1970s and 1980s, anesthesiologists were becoming interested in pain management. I remember an excellent conference I attended in San Francisco where I learned that anesthesiologists might well be the last resort for people with chronic pain; I always thought that was a very precarious position for a doctor to be in, so I didn't pursue pain management after doing some blocks, since my heart wasn't in it. Patients would start seeing an anesthesiologist after they were no longer helped by a psychiatrist. I liked to manage surgical pain and would do a lot of regional anesthesia even with people that were having a light general anesthetic.

Reno Medical Plaza

Outpatient surgi-centers and ambulatory surgical centers came into vogue in the mid 1970s, and I became involved in the first one in the area, Reno Medical Plaza (RMP). This was a brand new concept and I believe RMP was one of the first dozen, free-standing centers in the country. I helped design the building, the operating rooms, and helped bring it all together, along with Jan Pritchard, who subsequently married Dr. Tom Brady. Jan was a registered nurse, who had agreed to come on board. We ordered all the equipment, furniture, and instruments, and worked closely with the architect.

Dr. Carl Sauls, a Reno urologist, was the basic innovator of the surgi-center concept in Reno, and that came about as a result of a conflict he had with his landlord, Dr. Ken Maclean.[2] Ken was asked to renovate Saul's office on Ryland Street near Washoe Medical Center to incorporate a surgi-center, but he declined. Sauls then opened the new center. Dick Kaiser and I were asked to head up the anesthesia section, and we readily agreed to do that, but Dick backed out a little later, and I was there all by myself saying, "Oh, my God, now what am I going to do?"

I worked with the Associated Anesthesia Group from 1966 when I came to town and continued working there after the surgi-center opened. In fact, most of the doctors in the group rotated through the center. It became apparent in the early 1980s that the center needed full-time anesthesia coverage, as we became busy. Dr. Jack Flanary and I left the "big group," as it was known at that time. It was a friendly departure and we limited our practice to ambulatory surgery anesthesia at the Reno Medical Plaza. I remained there until my retirement in 1996.

Retirement

I have not practiced an anesthesia procedure since my retirement. Anesthesia frequently requires instantaneous "gut reactions" and one have to continuously monitor patients, even for minor procedures. I would listen to every breath they took during the surgery, and I could tell more from the way a patient was breathing than from a lot of the monitors I was using. An anesthesiologist's work is more of an art than a science, and I did not feel I could keep up my skills doing procedures on a part-time, hit-or-miss basis. I had worked a long time with Don Mousel and his very difficult pediatric cases. I just knew I could never continue doing that on less than a full-time basis, so I hung it up.

I retired in 1996 and figured I had had an enjoyable practice. I did not get all caught up in the less interesting aspects of practice, such as managed care, billing, and the headaches of running an office. I came into practice in the mid 1960s, about the time Medicare and Medicaid came into being, so I never really knew the completely free practice of medicine. I also never worried about whether I got paid or how much Medicare or Medicaid was paying; I left that up to the people in the front office. I knew that if I thought about it too much, I'd say, "Gee, I don't want to do this," so I found it easier just to say, "Bring them on, I'll do them all," and if I don't get paid, I don't even want to know about it because the ladies in the office will take care of it. I was aware, however, that managed care was changing things substantially.

I felt that government, in order to get those healthcare plans rolling, was initially very generous with their payments for Medicare and Medicaid services, and this made doctors and patients happy. In the years before, doctors were getting paid with a smile, a "Thank You," and occasionally a banana nut bread cake, or something like that. As the costs of medical care began going higher and higher, doctors became the villains for causing this increase, and they were the first to experience cuts in their fees.

My professional liability insurance took a big jump in the early 1970s and was up there at one time with the obstetricians and the neurosurgeons, but it began to come down and is now fairly reasonable. There were some big suits and settlements across the country about that time, but I think anesthesia has steadily become safer and safer. Suits have been infrequent in recent years and one of the reasons is that the advent of the laparoscope has reduced invasive procedures requiring deep anesthesia. Surgical instruments, I feel, will continue be get smaller and we'll see some procedures using intravascular technology.

Over the years new gases were touted and began showing up in operating rooms, but most were overrated. Each, however, moved the specialty forward a little bit and each was a little better than the last. Ether used to be our basic anesthetic agent and since then there has been a steady progression of agents, but there has been no "magic bullet," that miracle drug.

When I officially retired in 1996, I concentrated on doing some of the things I had put off doing over the years. I got interested in computers, and I built a house—a dream I had had for over twenty years. I drew up the plans, did the electrical work, laid tile and wood floors, hung cabinets, and pounded some nails. Our original plans called for the house to be built in Pleasant Valley, but we built in the Rosewood Lakes area, near Hidden Valley. The house took about two years to complete.

I really enjoyed my career in medicine and certainly enjoyed my choice of specialties, but was completely neutral when it came to giving advice to my children about what careers to follow. I wasn't against them going into medicine, but I remember my mom continuously urging me to be a doctor. She wasn't pushy, just firm, and this turned out to be the best thing in the world for me. I realize she knew what I didn't know at that time. I didn't follow her example and do that with my kids because, I guess, I resented being told what to do, even though it was in a loving way.

If I were to sum up my career in Reno, I think I would be proudest of the fact that I got the ambulatory surgi-center going. It wasn't a slam-dunk from the start—we struggled for the first few years, but it then took off. I think that was an innovation that was right for Reno and has proven to be right for the country.

Notes
[1] Dr. William Simpson was born in California in 1917 and licensed in Nevada in 1951. Dr. Robert Crosby was born in Ohio in and licensed in Nevada in 1949. Dr. Arthur Scott was born in 1918 and licensed in Nevada in 1948.

[2] Dr. Carl Sauls was born in 1926 and licensed and practiced urology in Nevada in 1961.

3: Dr. Theodore Berndt, Cardiology

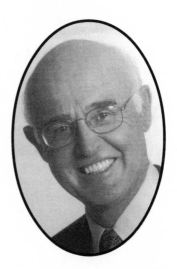

Dr. Theodore Berndt

Education

I was born April 6, 1940, in Argentina almost sixty-three years ago at the time of this writing and was number seven in line of ten children. We lived there until I was nine years old. My father, a Lutheran missionary, was furloughed to Portage, Wisconsin, and on extension of that furlough, we moved to Wausau, Wisconsin, where he became a minister of a church there. I grew up near Wausau, later graduating from high school in nearby Wittenberg.

Four of my brothers went into the ministry and that was a very politically correct profession for my family and for our times. One brother elected to become an engineer and one an economist, and, for various reasons, I decided to be of service by being a physician. I think I made that decision towards the end of my high school studies.

I'm not quite sure why I chose medicine but maybe it was something as simple as the encouragement of two high school friends who said they were going to be doctors. It certainly wasn't because there were lots of medical people in my family because there weren't any. It turned out that I was the only member of our family who had to make a living with my hands! All my brothers and sisters became scholars.

Medical Education and Residency

I enrolled in a premed program at the University of Wisconsin and entered the UW medical school at the end of my fourth year. On graduating,

I interned at Western Reserve in Cleveland and then went back to Wisconsin and did a two-year residency in internal medicine. I think it was during my time there that I decided to go into cardiology. Why? I think it was the exactness of cardiology that appealed to me, and I would say I was also greatly influenced by some excellent teachers. The name of one teacher at Wisconsin, Dr. George Rowe, comes to mind as the doctor who influenced me the most.

U.S. Army and Specialty Training

Then I went into the United States Army for two years serving at Camp Gordon in Augusta, Georgia. That part of the country was certainly different from Wisconsin, but I got used to the humidity and the heat and enjoyed my stay in the South quite a lot. Even though I had not completed my training in cardiology, I was allowed to do quite a lot in that area of medicine while at Camp Gordon; they even let me take care of Mamie Eisenhower when she was in town and, as everyone knows, President Eisenhower spent a lot of time on the Augusta national golf course.

When my military tour of duty was over, I decided to complete my cardiology training at Stanford University and was introduced to the West Coast. My brother lived in Palo Alto and that was a plus, but I chose Stanford because it had the reputation of being one of the best places, perhaps "the best" place in the country for cardiology studies at that time. I had two very good years there. On completion of my studies at Stanford, I was tempted to stay in academic medicine and almost returned to Wisconsin to be on staff at the medical school but elected to go into private practice instead. Interestingly, I wound up in a cardiology practice in New Orleans for my first two years out of fellowship. Dr. Charlie Steiner was doing some excellent work in heart catheterizations on the "West Bank" and I decided to join him; it was a very busy and rewarding two years for me. There was so much heart disease there. Everybody, it seemed, was fat and had coronary disease.

Cardiology in Reno

The Move to Reno

I was at a medical meeting in Kansas City in 1976 when I met Dr. Bob Barnet, who told me about an opportunity in Reno. Reno was very unusual in 1976; it was a good size community, but had no heart catheterization facilities. Bob, who had been in practice in Reno for several years, wanted an experienced cathing cardiologist to join him and to start the first cath lab at Washoe Medical Center. Initially I turned down the offer, but after thinking it over and remembering the wonderful experiences in the West at Stanford, I decided to join him. My leaving New Orleans did not mean I hadn't enjoyed my work there; it was just that I wasn't sure I wanted to relocate again so soon. This was a unique opportunity. I joined Bob and his associate, Jerry Zebrack, and, at almost the same time, my present associate, Richard Ganchan, also moved to Reno. There was another cardiologist who came to town in 1976 named Steve Savron who was recruited by internists Dave Roberts and Bob Myles.[1] That year saw an influx of three new cardiologists swelling the ranks from two to five new heart men in a short time.

Behind the Curve in Cardiology

In 1976 Bob Barnet had done a good job of establishing the concept of coronary care and telemetry units in this community, but Reno was somewhat behind the curve compared to other communities of this size in terms of invasive cardiology, heart catheterization, and heart surgery. The medical community had otherwise done a good job in attracting new equipment and technology in the other specialty areas.

Washoe Medical Center was clearly the hospital leader in cardiology technology in the mid 1970s, and Bob Barnet was involved in starting the first coronary care unit there. Since Bob was not a "cathing" cardiologist at that time, that procedure had to be done out of town: Sacramento, San Francisco, and Palo Alto. His interest in bringing the next level of coronary care to the area is the principle reason I am in Reno.

The First Cardiac Catheterization in Reno

I did the first cardiac catheterization in northern Nevada at Washoe Medical Center on Valentine's Day, February 14, 1977, on a lady named Mrs. Ethel Wright, and I remember it like it was yesterday. I had done several thousand by that time, but I was anxious for everything to go right this first time around and it went fine.

We received quite a bit of press coverage and after that, things went pretty fast. The area definitely needed heart surgery capability after that, and attempts were made by several groups to entice heart surgeons to town. Drs. Bob Nichols and Bill Keeler were actively trying to attract cardiac surgeons to town.[2] Dr. Nichols had training in heart surgery in the past and actually had a few cases referred to him by Dr. Savron. These doctors wanted to start the first heart surgery program for the area and there were some political battles fought. Our group did not get involved with referring to Dr. Nichols.

Cardiac Surgery

Dr. Barnet devoted his time and attention to recruiting a cardiac surgeon, Art Lurie, who arrived in Reno in 1978 and began doing by-pass procedures. Coronary artery bypass graft (CABG) exploded about that time. It started a whole new industry that just took off! Soon we were doing three to four hundred cases of open-heart surgery a year. That is the interesting part of the story. Prior to that time, the number of people sent out of the area for this procedure probably was only about one hundred, or possibly one hundred and fifty a year, but all at once three to four hundred cases were being done. Even after Dr. Lurie started his program, there were still a lot of patients being sent out of town, especially by physicians at St. Mary's Hospital. It soon became evident that physicians and administration at Saint's were not in full support of the cardiac surgery program at Washoe. The Washoe program was successful from the start and grew steadily over the next several years.

Steve Savron brought another cardiologist, Mike Newmark, to town in 1978 or 1979.[3] In 1980 Savron split off from the Roberts and Myles group. He started his own group and began a spirited competition between cardiologists.

Art Lurie took in a new partner, Dr. Bill Conran, in the early 1980s and they controlled cardiac surgery for quite a spell. Another heart surgeon came for a while, but he left after a short period. There were a few bumps on the cardiac surgery road, but they were more political than they were medical. Art Lurie was a very cautious and discreet surgeon, and I do not know of any medical setbacks in his surgery program. Dr. Bob Nichols' program was somewhat short lived, but he, too, was an excellent surgeon. One of the measures of acceptance of the cardiac surgery program in northern Nevada was the fact that numerous doctors and their family members were among the successful cases performed here rather than being referred elsewhere.

In the early 1990s, Drs. Kevin Linkus and Todd Chapman brought additional skills and training to the area, and the cardiac surgery program really prospered. Their coming coincided with the severe illness, multiple myeloma, suffered by Dr. Lurie. He and Dr. Conran later phased out their cardiac surgery practice and Dr. Lurie died in 1999.

Except for a few territorial fights, hospitals in Reno were very receptive to the work done by cardiologists in the area. They were receptive to buying new equipment and keeping up with staff training, as they understood the economic importance of quality cardiology and cardiac surgery programs in the area.

Washoe showed the first interest, developing the first cardiac cath lab, for example, but St. Mary's was quick to develop one and to begin their own cardiac surgery program. Administrators at Saint's recruited cardiologist Dr. Stan Thompson, who came in the early 1980s. He was later joined by others.

The county operated Washoe at the time, and I thought it was a beautiful hospital—very nice, clean, and well run. Carroll Ogren was an excellent administrator. He and Bob Barnet did good work in developing, funding, and staffing the cath lab and made a major contribution to the medical community. Although I never got to know Carroll personally, I felt he was an asset to the area. He assured everyone that Washoe would be the premier "high tech" and progressive hospital in the area and was always looking down the road ten to fifteen years. He was willing to spend whatever monies it would take to create an excellent lab, telemetry, and any other facility needed at the time. St. Mary's has always been a "high touch" center and it still is. I think that just comes with the territory—a Catholic hospital with sisters being so involved.

Reno's Nurses

I have always been impressed with the quality of nurses at Reno hospitals. There has been a lot of press in recent years about nurses being over-worked, under-appreciated, and under-paid, and I can understand those concerns. I think working conditions for nurses, while they have improved a good bit, still need more improvement. Salaries have definitely gone up, but nurses still feel they are stressed to the breaking point sometimes, and several have confided they can find less stressful jobs elsewhere. Many qualified young people who had originally thought of careers in nursing are now thinking about becoming doctors, and that option is certainly worth considering.

I do think educational requirements for nurses could be standardized, but still a nurse really becomes a good nurse after several years of practice and lots of training. Where they get that training and how they get it seems to be highly variable, but that is where a good nurse is molded. They are going through a very difficult period right now, and we are going to have a nursing shortage for many more years, but I know things will turn around.

To compound things, nurses have many other alternatives available to them besides just working in a hospital. In addition to a medical career, they can work for drug companies, home health programs, insurance and managed care companies; and this wealth of opportunity has naturally led to a shortage of nurses working directly with patients. That is the rub!

Cardiologists had no problem attracting nurses to work in the new cath labs when it first opened. They were well paid and were excited, but as time went on their excitement about cath lab work diminished due to consistently high stress levels and plain hard work. We have lost quite a few good nurses in the lab and have made extra efforts to attract and hold them.

Looking Back

I think back on the Reno medical community from time to time and marvel at how much it has grown. When I came here, there were no heart surgeons in the community. Intensive pulmonologists were just starting to come in. Neurologists were in relatively short supply, but we had an influx of well-trained doctors at that time, including Drs. Charlie Quaglieri and Mal Bacchus. We had excellent internists in Drs. Peter Rowe, J. Stephen Phalen, David Thompson, John Davis, and several others.[4] Generally, all other subspecialty areas were covered well.

There was a little resistance to the "new guys"—the cardiologists, coming on the Reno medical scene by some of the men who had been trained on-the-job to read electrocardiograms and other work. We were considered the new young "Turks" who had no experience, and it took some diplomacy, hard work, and some establishment of credentials before we were accepted, but it didn't take too long. I always felt I was readily accepted, but this was not the universal feeling of other cardiologists coming to town.

In the early days of my practice, I was obliged to do a lot of general medicine before restricting my practice to cardiology. Many of the new specialists coming to town had to conform to the culture of the practices they joined. I knew of one general surgeon who came to Reno and did sort of a general medicine practice for quite a period of time, until he could get his specialty practice going.

The Politics of Medicine

There was an active organized medical community in northern Nevada, but I stayed pretty much out of it for a long time. I just practiced medicine for five, eight, ten years, but after that, I started getting pulled into it—screaming and kicking. I have gotten involved more and more, but initially I felt the community had some icons that ran the political side of medicine: Bob Barnet, "Sal" Salvadorini, Ken Maclean, and Ernie Mack.[5] Medicine was run by these people—in one form or another—by their connections at the hospital, with the Nevada Board of Medical Examiners, and by involvement in workings of the Washoe County Medical Society. Reno was loaded with these few big icons and new doctors in town didn't argue with them; we just played their games. Things have changed over the years and that power has become much more diffused;

that concentration of medical-political power just doesn't exist anymore.

Ken Maclean was on the Nevada Board of Medical Examiners when I was up for Nevada licensure and that interview was very memorable! His oral examination questions had very little to do with medicine and were more of a "feeling out" process. He wanted to know who I was, what I wanted, and things like that. He also wanted me to know who "he" was. I always thought Ken was one of the good guys.

The University of Nevada School of Medical Sciences had just been converted to a four-year school and renamed the University of Nevada School of Medicine (UNSOM) when I came to Reno, and I thought at that time it was a "weak sister" of a medical school. There were politics being played between Washoe Medical Center and the medical school at that time, and I purposely stayed out of those battles. But early in my career I was a lecturer and our group served on the clinical staff at UNSOM. All of us today support the UNSOM cardiology program through lecturing and providing training for residents rotating through our services.

In the 1970s and 1980s there seemed to be a lot more interest in volunteering for things than today. Chief of medicine or chief of staff positions at our hospitals were sought after and doctors wanted that power and influence, but I am told that administrators today are having a tough time finding doctors willing to serve.

I guess I have shied away from a lot of medical-political offices over the years, but my partners have done excellent work here. For example, Dick Ganchan was chief of staff at Washoe Medical Center about a dozen years ago—a position I have successfully avoided. Other positions I have not actively sought were president of the Washoe County Medical Society and the Nevada State Medical Association. Another of my partners, John Williamson, will be president of the state association this year and is serving as chief of staff at St. Mary's Regional Medical Center. This is not to say that I haven't paid my dues. I have been on the Washoe Medical Center Board of Directors for many years, and for the last six or seven years, I have served on the board of Washoe Health System (WHS). WHS is the parent corporation for the medical center, the Hometown Health Program health maintenance organization (HMO), and a number of other subsidiaries.

Advances in Cardiology

The most important advances in my field during my career had to be the introduction of ultrasound technology (echocardiography) and the coming of age of intervention cardiology (angiography) with the placement of balloons and stents. Angioplasty procedures started in the mid to late 1980s and really soared; undoubtedly those were the biggest advances that have occurred in cardiology and they were revolutionary to the sub-specialty. Echocardiography, or ultrasound, was taught to a very limited extent when I was in training at Stanford, but angioplasty and stents, of course, were never taught at all, so I had to learn most of that when I got into practice.

Dr. Donald Spring was also well trained in this new technology, and when he came to the area, we worked together on the first angioplasty program at Washoe. I give him credit for his leadership in advancing angioplasty and stenting in this community more than anybody else.

There have been many excellent pharmaceuticals—whole new classes of drugs, put on the market during my career, that have been invaluable in treating hypertension. We treat heart failure differently because of these new drugs and procedures, and we treat heart attacks in entirely new ways: we go after them—we attack them. By quickly opening the blocked vessels with thrombolytic agents or with angioplasty, we have been highly successful in saving lives. Those things didn't even exist when I got off the train years ago. We have incredibly good tools now compared to twenty to thirty years ago.

If one looks at the literature, there has been a dramatic decrease in the number of cardiac deaths per age group, and that can be accredited to new drugs, procedures, and medical management. People are still dying, of course, but what we are preventing is premature cardiovascular disease, and we have made a lot more progress than cancer prevention, for example. But thirty to forty years ago there were a lot of people who were dying of heart attacks in their fifties and sixties, and that is much, much less likely to happen today. Deaths due to heart attacks occur now when people are seventy-five, eighty, or eighty-five years old. That's excellent progress.

Years ago, people with heart attacks were in the hospital for extended stays, on bed rest for months, and had lingering disabilities; that has totally changed. We now treat heart attacks very aggressively up front. Patients are out of the hospital in three to four days and usually go home with a stent or angioplasty; they are back to work within two to three weeks.

Without a doubt, I believe that cardiology is one of the subspecialties that has made the most progress in the last twenty-five to thirty years and lives have been greatly extended.

Preventive cardiology is the apple pie, the motherhood of cardiology, but people don't want to invest in it. The public has been slow to comprehend the benefits of prevention. They seem to want a quick fix, a simple pill, but that is not the answer to preventing heart disease. All the medical procedures and pharmaceuticals on the scene today have come about because preventative cardiology has not been practiced. Coronary artery disease is highly preventable. While doctors emphasize that only the affluent and some of the upper middle classes in our society practice coronary disease prevention, the problem is that most of the middle and lower classes, and some ethnic groups, are very negligent in terms of following risk factor modification. They are overweight, don't exercise, don't watch their diets, and smoke. Yes, they smoke! That is the biggest risk factor of all—that is the big answer—we have all the evidence we need.

Challenges in Cardiology

I think one of the biggest challenges in cardiology today is the well-known fact that practicing good cardiology is expensive. It is expensive because it is so technology intensive and a valid question arises: How much is society willing to spend? We are hitting the wall today in the expense of saving lives threatened by coronary disease and heart attacks. Defibrillators have the potential of benefiting huge numbers of people— that benefit can be incredible. We now know we can extend life at least a year for a lot of these people, but can we do that for all of these people at a cost that can exceed $50,000, $60,000, or $70,000 per patient?

I think gene therapy for certain diseases is coming down the pike. I think we will be able to manipulate that, but that's still a ways off, and I don't think cardiologists in Reno will be getting involved soon. We will refer to centers elsewhere. It is in such an infancy stage. I think one of the biggest things that is going to happen in the next five years is the development of the super stents. Stents that we now place in patients re-close in about six months time in twenty to thirty percent of the cases. These new super stents being evaluated by the FDA basically have no re-stenosis rate. They are predicting that, with this new technology, five years from now we will only be doing half of the heart surgery we are doing now. So, we will be placing a lot more stents and doing much less surgery.

If these new stents begin replacing old stents that clog up, it would reduce the need for most of the coronary bypass surgery being performed. Big heart surgery programs around the country that have spent so much money on buildings, expensive cath labs, and operating suites could be looking at some rocky financial times down the road.

Shortage of Cardiologists

Another problem I see on the horizon will be a shortage of practicing and academic cardiologists. Training programs are shrinking because of lack of funding. Then too, a lot of cardiologists are retiring early, in their fifties and early sixties, because they have done so well financially the past several years. Also the demand for their services with all this new technology keeps exploding. Many feel they simply can't keep up the frantic pace. Nobody predicted this. Headhunters tell us that orders for cardiologists are the most difficult to fill.

There is no quick fix to solving the cardiologist shortage problem. Our national specialty society has been looking into it through various manpower task forces, but a big problem seems to be in finding adequate funding for training programs. Once there is a shortage, it takes eight to ten years to fix it.

Looking down the road I sometimes think about retiring, but I don't think it is in the cards for me any time soon. Cardiology is hard work and there have been plenty of times I would like to ease up on the long hours, night calls, and weekend work, and I may do that within the next year or two, but I plan to work for quite a few more years yet. I really enjoy what I am doing. Reno is been an excellent place to live, work, and raise my family. The medical community is top notch, and our hospitals are truly state of the art.

Notes
[1] Dr. David Roberts was born in 1931 and licensed in Nevada in 1963.

[2] Dr. Nichols did the first open-heart surgery in Reno on Dale Hart. Drs. William Keeler and Robert Simon assisted Dr. Nichols.

[3] Dr. Steve Savron was born in 1942 and licensed in Nevad a in 1976.

[4] Dr. Peter Rowe was born in Montana in 1912 and was licensed in Nevada in 1948.Dr. Steven Phalen was born in South Dakota in 1919 and was licensed in Nevada in 1952. Dr. David Thompson was born in Ohio in 1923 and was licensed in Nevada in 1955.

[5] Dr. Vasco A. Salvadorini was born in California in 1915 and was licensed in Nevada in 1950.

4: Dr. Roderick Sage, Dermatology

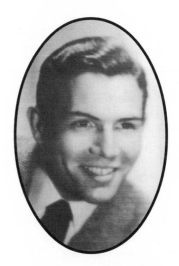

Dr. Roderick Sage

Family Tradition in Medicine

When my son, Dr. Jonathan Garey-Sage graduated from the University of Nevada School of Medical Sciences in 1984, he became the fourth generation Sage to earn an M.D. degree. This became possible with the advent of our medical school, and we have been delighted to have him settled in a successful urologic practice in Reno. These four generations of physicians have collectively witnessed a monumental progression of medical science, spanning well over a century.

Jonathan's great-grandfather was Fred Carlton Sage, M.D., an 1893 graduate of the School of Medicine at the University of Iowa. Fred first practiced in Hudson, Iowa after graduation; this was a tiny rural community from which he moved, after several years, to nearby Waterloo. Soon he obtained advanced training in eye, ear, nose, and throat in New York City and Chicago. He practiced in that specialty in Waterloo and, until his retirement at age ninety, from his practice in San Pedro, California, to which he had relocated in 1928.

My father, Erwin Carlton Sage, M.D., graduated in 1924 from the medical school at Iowa. He interned for a year in obstetrics and gynecology and then did general practice until 1936 in Eagle Grove, a northern Iowa community of 4000. This was the time of the Great Depression, the stresses of which ultimately induced him to obtain a fellowship to the Johns Hopkins School of Public Health and Hygiene, from which he earned a Master of Public Health degree in 1937. This was followed by a productive eleven years as director of the Des Moines County Health

Department in Burlington, Iowa.

Erwin served in the U.S. Navy Medical Corps during WW II. His most significant duty was as chief medical officer on an attack transport, the USS *Mifflin* "APA 207" during the Iwo Jima and Okinawa campaigns.

In May of 1948 he became assistant director of the San Francisco Health Department. In 1960, at that department's mandatory retirement age, he "retired" to a new and rewarding career as superintendent of the Nampa State School and Hospital in Idaho. This institution, which cared for retarded patients, had fallen sadly behind times; in fact, it belonged to the dark ages. Through certain perseverance, he hauled it out by its heels into the bright daylight, turning it into a vibrant, high-level school for disadvantaged citizens. He further capped this career by developing a masterfully planned and staffed hospital facility.

My mother's (Katherine Sage) contribution to his endeavor was to organize a women's auxiliary in Nampa and nearby Boise for the state school. For the foyer of the new hospital, named the "Erwin C. Sage, M.D. Memorial Hospital," she selected a fitting inscription taken from Matthew 25:40: "For inasmuch as you have done unto one of the least of these my brethren, you have done it unto me."

Erwin's tenure at the state school ended in 1967, but he continued in other work in the area, first as director of the nearby Canyon County Health Department. For three years he served as an inspector-consultant for an AMA regional hospital survey team, and finally was the blood bank physician in Nampa.

Mother's distinguished career in volunteer activities, marked by upper-level service in the League of Women Voters and Salvation Army in Iowa, California, and Idaho ended, as did Erwin's, in the late 1970s. They both died within a few months of each other in 1984 and 1985.

My dad had been in practice in Eagle Grove for only eight months, when I was born February 13, 1926. My brother, Fred, had preceded me by eighteen months. He had joined an older, legendary country physician, Dr. Charles Morse, who had been in Eagle Grove almost since it first became a town. Erwin left Dr. Morse to open his own practice after a couple of years.

We enjoyed good times until 1930 when the Depression arrived in full force. Jobs were lost, banks failed, there were farm commodity wars about the state, and everywhere there was a striking sense of despair. But folks continued to get sick, babies arrived, and people died. The money faucet went dry. Despite this, we got along quite well. Bills were paid with the barter system. We ate beef, poultry, pork, and fresh vegetables. Necessary services, such as, housework and laundry, were furnished by the wives or mothers of some of Erwin's patients. My older brother Fred and I were enrolled in a weekly tap dance class taught by a patient in return for Dad's delivering her baby. That ended, however, when she announced that we were to participate in a tap dance recital.

Erwins' office was on the second floor of the downtown Wassom Building, the stairs of which I swept every Saturday morning. The reward was 10¢, to which was added a weekly allowance of 15¢: the total—two-bits (or, two candy bars, one ice cream cone, and a Hoot Gibson cowboy show at Ed Morris' movie palace, "The Princess"). We lived in a comfortable six-room home that rented for $30 a month, paid 18¢ for a gallon of gas, and could buy a new Chevy or Ford for $600. At that rate, who needed a big wad of cash!

As a youngster, I was able to observe what a medical practice was like. It was tough work, compounded by hard times. Dad's interest in obstetrics added to his burden, since many of his deliveries were out in the country in all sorts of weather, reached by roads that were poorly kept, to say the least. My medical career started in dad's office, watching him do tonsillectomies, remove wens from the scalp, and suture lacerations.

He must have felt a sense of frustration and helplessness in the face of killer and crippling diseases, such as diphtheria, typhoid fever, tuberculosis, pneumonia, and whooping cough, even though immunization programs were available. Certainly this was long before the advent of antibiotics. The nearest hospital was in Fort Dodge, Iowa, thirty miles away, and in mid-winter with unpaved, unplowed roads, it might as well have been on the moon. This situation sparked his interest in public health.

For a solo practitioner, as Erwin was then, weekends could be a bear. He treated patients all day Saturday. Since it was the farmers' day in town, he saw them until midnight or one A.M. in his office. Then on Sunday morning he held more office hours. In a small town like Eagle Grove everyone knew where we lived, so Sunday afternoon curbside visits at our home were commonplace.

In spite of this, Erwin had time for other interests. He became the local commander of the American Legion, which was, at that time, a major national patriotic and political organization. He was elected to the school board, ultimately as president, and every fall he was the doctor for the Eagle Grove High School football team, the Eagles. Golf became a pastime for all of us. We joined the local country club, took lessons, and played once or twice a week.

By 1936, after eleven years of this general practice grind, Erwin realized that the rewards no longer outweighed the sacrifices. This led to his year at Johns Hopkins School of Public Health. We enjoyed our time in Baltimore, and were able to soak up the history and culture of the East long before the population and development explosion altered the face of the area.

We returned to Iowa in 1937 when Erwin was appointed the director of the Des Moines County Public Health Department in Burlington. This was an old Mississippi River town of twenty-five thousand souls, which had its own charm and interest.

His first task was to convince the city fathers that a milk ordinance was of the utmost urgency. When it became effective, by law, all the milk sold in Burlington had to be pasteurized. Immediately, the incidence of enteric diseases dropped, and Erwin became a local hero. In due time, he started programs to control mosquitoes (and malaria), fostered immunization and vaccination clinics, and worked to eradicate venereal diseases, among others.

Education

As I entered Burlington High School, there was no question about my going into medicine—I knew nothing else, and there was no family business for me to inherit. Indeed, brother Fred was in the same boat; he later became a hospital administrator. After the usual stints of high school football, writing for the school paper, and appearing in a few school plays, we all went off to the war in the spring and summer of 1943. Erwin went into the navy medical corps, beginning his duties in Bainbridge, Maryland; Fred and I went into the V-12 program. This was a college training program to prepare young men to be naval officers.

U.S. Navy

I was assigned to Notre Dame University in the V-12 premed program. After a couple of marginal and less than marginal semesters, this episode came to a merciful end. At that time, I was about as ready to pursue a fruitful college premedical program as I was to play quarterback for the Chicago Bears. There was some redemption after boot camp when I became an electronics technician; however, my most satisfying effort was as the editor of the newspaper "The Nereid," of the Submarine Tender *USS Nereus* "AS 17."

By the end of my service in 1946, I had begun to "gel," and fate granted me another chance to cut the mustard. My new motivation level and attitude helped me do well at the University of Iowa as an undergraduate in premed. The experience at Notre Dame made me realize the importance of allowing youngsters a few years, if needed, to mature (The Mormons deal with this situation by sending their nineteen year-olds on two-year church missions).

Medical School and Residency

I entered the freshman medical school class at Stanford in 1949, finishing in 1953. From there I interned at the Medical College of Virginia (MCV), then had a year of medical residency at Dartmouth. I returned West to Stanford Hospital in San Francisco for three years of dermatology residency with Dr. Eugene Farber, one of the bright young professors in our field at that time.

Jackie Price and I were married in 1952. By the time we finished the dermatology program in 1958, we had two handsome sons, Jonathan and Jeff. Son Rowan arrived in September of 1958, while the youngest brother, Andrew, joined us in February of 1962.

It was time to find a place to put down roots and get to work. In searching about for a suitable community, we briefly inspected the bay area and Sacramento. Dr. George Kulchar, one of our wise and practical consultants at Stanford, suggested that we take a look at Reno. He said, "You don't want to go to Sacramento. That's a cow town. Reno is where the action is."

Reno Dermatology

Move to Reno

So, Reno it became. Jackie and I drove up to Reno over Memorial Day weekend in 1958; found a house to rent on South Arlington Avenue, and a new office (still unfinished) at 580 West Fifth Street. I took the state board oral exams and found the several examiners to be most congenial.

Thanks to Dr. Roland Stahr this all fell into place. He had practiced pediatrics in Ft. Dodge, Iowa near our hometown of Eagle Grove. When I was eleven, he helped me through a bout of poliomyelitis. Roland and Dudley, his wife, moved to Reno in 1940 and we lost track of them, but reconnected when I became interested in coming to Reno. Roland was truly an important figure in Reno. He was acclaimed as Nevada's Outstanding Doctor and was elected to the presidency of the Nevada State Medical Society in 1965. He was a dear friend and counselor who was most helpful in getting us started in practice and in the community. His advice for me to remain independent was excellent, and I avoided involvement with any particular group, allowing me to take referrals from all camps.

For the first two months of practice I used Roland's office at Sierra and California Streets; then I moved over to 580 West Fifth. These offices were basically designed for dentists, but with a bit of modification, mine suited me very well. There were two treatment rooms and a central lab space. I installed my ultraviolet light in one room and, after lining the walls with lead, put my new Picker x-ray in the other room. We used a lot of superficial x-ray for skin cancers, chronic dermatoses, and sometimes for acne. The ultraviolet light was also useful for some of those same problems. Both modalities have long since been phased out because of the now well-recognized hazards with ionizing radiation.

When I arrived in Reno, I made an effort to get around, shake hands, and say "howdy" to as many colleagues as would see me—even in Susanville and Carson City. One lovely autumn day in 1958 I rode the Union Pacific train out to Elko to attend my first state medical convention. Dr. Wes Hall, who had started through the chairs enroute to the AMA presidency, was a most cordial host, as was Nelson Neff, the society's executive secretary. After sitting in on a few lectures, devouring a delicious western barbecue, and shaking many hands, I thought to myself, "Boy, did I luck out."

I became busy and was soon building a bank account. In fact, about five months later, my accountant surprised me with the news that I owed a bundle for taxes. So, I took out a loan and acquired a new accountant.

We found a very pleasant woman, Mrs. Brown, to help us with the household chores and baby tending, and I hired a delightful office secretary-nurse. The following spring though she abandoned ship—both her marriage and mine. At this point, I launched the "longest continuing search" for office help in history. I could feel my heart sink when I arrived at work on several Monday mornings with the door still locked, lights out, and three or four patients dancing about, from one foot to the other, wondering, "Where is the doc?" Fortunately, Jackie was able to come down and bail me out, but then the frantic quest for a new "girl" would start. Finally, Bessie Williams arrived on the scene and served me well for twenty-six years until she succumbed to a stroke in 1987.

It was four years before Jackie and I managed any major traveling. The first trip was to the International Congress of Dermatology in Washington, D.C. in 1962, but I frequently attended the San Francisco Dermatologic Society's monthly meetings. I found that the local gatherings of the Washoe County Medical Society, Reno Surgical Society, and Nevada State Medical Society meetings were excellent and pertinent. Sometime later, with the turmoil related to health care problems, the county, and state meetings became quite politically oriented, causing some of us to lose interest in organized medicine.

By 1963 my space at 580 West Fifth Street seemed to shrink. Major expansion was underway at 975 Ryland, and I wrangled myself an invitation to move there just in time to plan my space as I wanted it. The most useful addition was a big skylight in each of three treatment rooms.

975 Ryland Street Office

I always considered 975 Ryland to be the premium location in Reno. Drs. Peter Rowe, Steve Phalen, and David Thompson were down the hall in medicine; Ken Maclean, William Tappan, and Donald Guisto were across the hall in surgery; Jim Greer, Chuck Lanning, and later, Don Mousel, were nearby in ophthalmology, while Bob Myles, Lowell Peterson, and Don Mohler had offices in their respective specialties.[1] We had excellent lab and pharmacy services. Shortly afterwards, the building at 890 Mill opened, as did the 1000 Ryland facility. We were certainly in the center of things—Washoe hospital was a five-minute walk, St. Mary's was a ten-minute drive—both were congenial places to admit patients or to consult. I usually had one or two in-hospital patients until the cost of such care became prohibitive.

My arrival in Reno in 1958 doubled the number of skin specialists in town. Dr. Mort Falk had been in Reno since 1952, though Dr. Charles McNitt practiced in Reno for a while during the 1950s.[2] Mort and I enjoyed a friendly relationship for many years. He employed several associates during the 1970s, particularly Tom Standlee, then Alan McCarty, and finally Steve Billstein. In the years when he was solo, he was very busy. It helped me immensely to be able to see some of his overflow of patients.

When the new University of Nevada medical school opened in 1971 as a two-year facility, Mort and I organized a weeklong dermatology course for the students, almost covering the whole field. Perhaps this was too much for them, but we figured it would be the only exposure they would have to skin diseases. The medical school expanded to the four years in 1978, and we adjusted by spreading our teaching material into the third and fourth years. Mort and I also participated in a dermatology-teaching clinic at the Reno VAMC, where we saw patients weekly until the unending VA hassles forced us to abandon this enterprise.

Consultant to Student Health

My most satisfying outside work has been to serve as consultant to the UNR Student Health Service. I started there shortly after Dr. Bob Locke left the directorship, to be followed by Dr. Joe Beres.[3] We expanded the S.H.S. from almost-adequate space in Juniper Hall to the sparkling and roomy clinic in the Nell J. Redfield Building, adjacent to the medical school. This has numerous treatment rooms, a full-time and well-trained professional staff, and plenty of patients.

Starting a brand new practice in 1958 was a challenge and an adventure. After nine years of preparation, beginning at Stanford in 1949, I figured I must know almost everything about dermatology. Pretty soon

I realized that there were a few gaps and crevasses in my knowledge of the skin, but with continued effort these began to fill in.

Advances in Dermatology

I introduced the use of liquid nitrogen to the community for the treatment of many skin lesions—from warts to superficial skin cancers. This beat dry ice by a mile. We were using five fluorouracil (5FU) topically to treat pre-malignant growths. Our use of oral antibiotics, especially the tetracyclines for acne, was expanding, but we had to be cautious about side effects, such as sun sensitization. It was another thirty years before we concluded that chocolate and a few other foods were highly overrated as troublemakers. We had a number of systemic and topical steroids available to treat a great variety of inflammatory diseases, and drug company detail reps were hard at our heels to make sure we knew all about the latest and greatest developments.

Psoriasis was then, and still is, a great bugaboo: a miserable ailment to have, and frustrating to treat. When people say, "Doc, your patients never die and they never get well," they are talking about psoriasis. New and frightfully expensive medications are becoming available to treat this and other tough problems, but there remains a long road to travel before psoriasis is routinely controlled. The best newer drug is 13-cis Retinoic Acid ("Accutane") for the care of severe acne. It has significant side effects, especially in relation to pregnancy, but does it ever work.

The American Academy of Dermatology has become a leading force in dermatologic research, educational programs for doctors and lay people, and promotion of a multitude of preventative projects. A few of its goals are: (1) to elucidate the dangers of sun exposure, (2) to sponsor screening clinics nationwide for skin cancer and especially melanoma, (3) to promote investigations and reporting on a large number of immunologic disorders, including contact allergies, through such agencies as the Dermatology Foundation.

When I joined the academy in 1958, there were about twelve hundred members. At our annual meeting in March 2003, sixteen thousand registrants were present. In 1958 we had one significant journal, *The Archives of Dermatology*. Now, there are perhaps a dozen high quality journals. The annual convention of the academy is renowned as one of the premier teaching-learning meetings in all of medicine and its scope is international.

The expansion of dermatology has led to a variety of problems—growing pains, perhaps. A few years back it was considered to be unethical for doctors to advertise; a business card printed in a publication of one sort or another was about the extent of it. Now, with the advertising media hard at work, television, newspapers, magazines, and even telephone books all carry what I consider to be distasteful and garish full-page, full-color ads extolling the skills and virtue of the practitioner. I may be old fashioned, but this goes against the grain, and it certainly indicates a major shift in our mores. Medicine as a noble profession suffers because of this.

The emergence of the cosmetic dermatologist is a complex relationship between service and the financial reward. In some cases, these doctors charge big fees, cash on the barrelhead, for procedures that insurance companies scoff at. Laser surgery, for example, has its place and is becoming more useful; however, if you put all of that money into a laser machine, you jolly well have to use it a lot in order to pay for it. Mohs' surgery for malignant skin lesions, in the proper hands, is a marvelous technique and falls into a different category, fulfilling a distinct need for care not available otherwise. Botox injections to flatten out wrinkles are inordinately costly and frequently effective for no more than six to eight months. I wonder, with all of this cosmetic stuff going on— much of it frivolous—who is going to treat the poor devil with his intractable pruritus or generalized erythroderma? There is an unfortunate rift between the surgical and medical dermatologists, which, I fear, will deepen over time. Some of this relates to the insurance reimbursement schedules for surgical procedures, which, compared to the medical procedures, are considerably greater.

Everything in sight has become more expensive: the cost of a medical education has skyrocketed, the cost of running an office is burdensome, as are all forms of medical-related insurance. Our fees have had to increase commensurately.

The price of medication has risen inordinately—partly because the traffic will bear it—but after being annoyed to death with television drug advertising, I suspect those drug costs are at least doubled to pay for the ads. These represent enormous drug company advertising budgets, and, I think, are totally unnecessary. A doctor should be able to prescribe the medication he thinks is appropriate without being badgered to write for some drug the patient saw promoted in a TV ad.

Reno has grown by leaps and bounds since 1958. The medical community, likewise, is expanding. From the two of us—Dr. Falk and myself—in dermatology at that time, we now have over fifteen skin specialists in our area, plus a few itinerants who come and go without putting down roots or contributing to the community.

Since arriving in Reno forty-five years ago, Jackie, our sons, and I have enjoyed a delightful life. Medicine and dermatology have been stimulating and rewarding. I have developed worthy professional and personal relationships with many of my fellow physicians. We have been able to marvel at and participate in the astounding advances in the medical sciences. Our pride in the University of Nevada School of Medicine is well deserved, and it is gratifying to realize that many of us have helped it to become an excellent institution.

It has been my joy to awaken each morning and literally or figuratively shake hands with myself that we have lived in Reno these many years and practiced dermatology and medicine. Certainly, this has been the best of both worlds. I have been asked, over the years, to assess my greatest accomplishment in life. Without hesitating, I answer that it has been for Jackie and me to raise and nurture our four sons. Getting them through the turbulence of growing up, educating them, and guiding them into fulfilling careers has been totally satisfying. The fact that they all turned out to be exceptional lads, I hope, reflects on both of us as good parents. We continue to maintain our close relationships with the boys and with their growing families.

Finally, in looking over the span of time from those hard-bitten, tight-lipped Depression years in Northern Iowa, to the abundance of Reno in 2003, there comes an awareness of the phenomenal changes in medicine, and everything else in our world. It has been, and continues to be, an amazing, startling, and always fascinating adventure of the most unique sort.

Notes
[1] Dr. William Tappan, a general surgeon, graduated form the Univ. of Mich. in 1945 and was licensed in Nevada in 1952. Dr. Lowell Peterson, a general surgeon, graduated from the Univ. of Minn. in 1938 and licensed in Nevada in 1952.

[2] Dr. Charles McNitt was born in Mich. in 1896 and licensed in Nevada in 1946.

[3] Dr. Robert Locke was born in Utah in 1920 and licensed in Nevada in 1946.

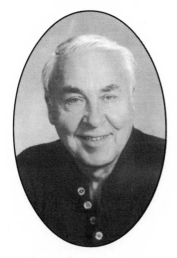

Dr. John M. Davis

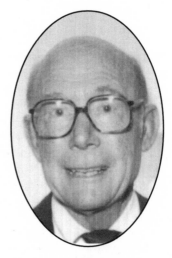

Dr. Frank E. Roberts

5: Internal Medicine

Dr. John M. Davis

Education

I was born January 31, 1928, in Chicago and shortly afterwards my family moved to Oklahoma, where we lived for six years. In 1935 we migrated to Santa Ana, California along with Henry Fonda and lots of other people. Both of my parents were physicians who trained at Rush Medical College at the University of Chicago. My mother was a pediatrician who stayed home during those years in Oklahoma. She began her practice of pediatrics in Santa Ana and my father was the first urologist in Orange County. I had nothing but total exposure to medicine as I grew up. We would sit at the dinner table and talk about the medical events of the day. I could never have considered anything but being a doctor; it was ingrained in me. My sister, with the same exposure, however, chose a career in interior design after graduating from University of California, Berkeley.

I finished high school in Santa Ana and began my undergraduate education in 1945 at Stanford University. I earned my A.B. and M.D. degrees at Stanford, got married while there, and after an internship at San Francisco City and County Hospital, I went into the air force.

U.S. Air Force and Residency

Those of us in the study of medicine had been deferred from the draft during the period of time we were in school on the contingency that we owed the government two years of military service after graduating. I was stationed at Warren Air Force Base in Cheyenne, Wyoming, for two very interesting years, 1956-'57—what a good experience. Dr. Charles Rammelcamp, the famous physician from Cincinnati and Cleveland areas, ran the Streptococcal Disease Laboratory. Studies were on going in streptococcal diseases, rheumatic fever, and nephritis, and I had the great experience of running the rheumatic fever ward for a year.

When my air force hitch was up, I returned to San Francisco and went into an internal medicine residency back at the city and county hospital. I had a great professor named J. K. Lewis. I then went across town to Stanford Lane Hospital and did my second year in internal medicine. As one of my colleagues who joined me for that move said, "We moved from the hairy armpit school of medicine to the magnolia and moonlight school of medicine." After a year there, I took a fellowship in cardiopulmonary diseases for my third year of training. The year was 1959 and it was time to leave the area. My wife and I realized we did not like the urban sprawl going on in the San Francisco and Orange County areas. Since we had friends in northern Nevada, Dr. Rod Sage and his wife Jackie, and had come to enjoy skiing in Wyoming and the magnificent outdoors, both of which were available in Reno, along with great fishing and a beautiful community, the decision was quickly made to relocate to northern Nevada. We have never regretted it.

Internal Medicine in Reno (Davis)

Move to Reno

When I got to Reno, I was quite interested in learning all I could about the quality of facilities, the level of medical technology, and meeting and talking with as many physicians as possible. I had trained at a good university and I naturally had certain expectations as far as what to look for in support services, laboratory, radiology, and the level of training of local physicians. Also, both hospitals were pretty well up to speed in most of the things I would need to practice quality internal medicine, so that was never a problem. I quickly became impressed with the quality of physicians who practiced here; the surgeons and other medical specialists were top-notch. That quality has been maintained the entire time I have been here. The area has been blessed with very well trained physicians and I guess they have been attracted here because it is such a great place to live and raise a family. The people here are well rounded and motivated toward things that expand life experiences.

Cardiology in Reno

In those early days, even with my special training in cardiology, there really wasn't much I could do on the community level as far as developing a specialty cardiac laboratory and that type of thing. That opportunity didn't really materialize for the community until some ten to fifteen years later. After moving to Reno and establishing my practice, I became a primary referral person for doctors whose patients had a heart attack (myocardial infarction). I took care of most of them in the community. I did a lot of general internal medicine practice and, as time evolved in my thirty-five year practice, my patients grew older and a lot of them developed significant cardiac problems along the way.

Well, technology was moving right along too, and I recall cardiac pacemakers appearing in the 1960s. I identified a couple of patients who had near complete heart block and were having fainting spells and near-death episodes from their hearts almost stopping. They were candidates for pacemakers, and those were not yet available in Reno.

In the mid to late 1960s, as I began seeing more and more extremely sick cardiac patients, I would refer them to Stanford since I had a lot of contacts down there. When they got back from Stanford with their permanent pacemakers, they had many years of enjoyable life afterwards.

The same thing was occurring with valve surgery. I referred a number of patients who had rheumatic valvular heart disease and other types of heart involvement requiring surgery. When they reached the critical point in their disease process where they needed surgery, off to Stanford they'd go as that procedure simply was not available here and would not be available until the late 1970s. So, there was a period of over fifteen years when we had to handle that type of cardiac patient by shipping them out of town. Then things changed. Management of seriously ill cardiac patients changed.

Cardiac Intensive Care Unit (CICU) at WMC

The Cardiac Intensive Care Unit opened at Washoe Medical Center and we were able to manage heart attack patients here in town. When patients were admitted with a myocardial infarction, there wasn't a whole lot we could do for them other than manage the complications of abnormal heart rhythm and congestive heart failure with drugs. That is what we did. We didn't have much in the way of monitoring equipment, but our management included maintaining the patient in the hospital often for two weeks after the end of the heart attack.

The following excerpt is from *People Make the Hospital: The History of Washoe Medical Center*:

> "Dr. Peter Rowe started cardiology at Washoe Medical Center and Reno shortly after he arrived in 1948. He was trained in internal medicine and cardiology at the University of Michigan.... ...January 1963...Joanne Wessel, RN was appointed manager of beds where patients with heart disease were admitted. ...The next step in cardiology came after Dr. Bernie Lown, a colleague of Dr. George Smith's from Boston visited Reno. He had established the first cardiac intensive care unit in the country at the Peter Bent Brigham Hospital. ...he recommended that Washoe Medical Center build a CICU. As a result Washoe Medical Center's CICU was the second or third unit in the country. ...[WMC's unit] opened in September 1965...."

Then invasive techniques became more available in the management of people in the Cardiac Intensive Care Units and the regular Intensive Care Units. The Swan-Ganz catheter, which is introduced through the subclavian vein into the right side of the heart and into the pulmonary circulation, became available. Pressures could now be measured and treatment could be refined to the point where we were able to respond not only to how the patient looked, but also to what these pressures were, and we could adjust medications as a consequence. I learned to do that in the early to mid-1970s.

This also involved using arterial lines, which are catheters inserted into the radial artery to continuously monitor the patient's blood pressure. So, we had circulation management in both the right and left sides of the heart. We were able to monitor acutely ill patients in a much more specific fashion with these tools than ever before. These modalities, the Swan-Ganz catheter and arterial lines, permitted us to not only manage cardiac patients, but also other acutely ill patients as well. People in shock for whatever reasons were given medicines to counteract whatever was going on that was detrimental to their blood circulation. Drs. Gene Kalin and Paul Gregory, who were Reno anesthesiologists, helped me learn arterial line technology and gave me on-the-job training long before invasive cardiologists came to town. I learned the Swan-Ganz procedure when I began putting in pacemakers. In my fellowship at Stanford I did work in the dog laboratory where we actually inserted catheters into dogs to do scientific measurements.

Beginning Practice

Not long after I came to town I was introduced to Dr. Fred Elliott, who had been in Reno for probably seven or eight years and was interested in having someone join him in his internal medicine practice.[1] He was located on St. Lawrence Avenue and we shared office space and call time. While we were never business partners, our association was a very good arrangement. We worked awfully hard in those days, as on-call responsibilities were tremendous. We each carried the responsibilities of our own patients all week, then Fred and I would cover for each other on alternate weekends. Those were extremely busy weekends because we provided coverage for two practices. When our weekends off came around, we basically spent those days recovering from the fifteen straight days of continuous work.

I never did a practice comparison, but I had a very large practice in those early days. There weren't many of us who were doing internal medicine in town, and we were relied upon by all the other general practitioners and surgeons who had need of our skills. It involved a lot of hospital medicine. The other thing was that our on-call coverage at Washoe Medical Center emergency room came up pretty regularly. In other words, the emergency room was set up so that we had twenty-four hour calls three or four times each month in medicine, surgery, orthopedics, and all the various specialties. If an emergency room patient was ill with a medical problem, we were called in to determine what to do with him—whether to admit for treatment, or treat and release. And this was done for no fee from the patient or hospital. That is completely different from the way it is done now. We just considered it a part of our duty and our responsibility. Reno was a stopping-over place for travelers going across the country and for others who had come here to gamble. Many times they would wind up in the hospital, which meant they had no personal physician in the area. Californians would come here and many of them would stay up all night drinking and pass out in the casinos. They would be hauled to Washoe Medical Center emergency room by ambulance. Some had just over-extended themselves and just needed some temporary treatment, and some were sick enough to be admitted. It is amazing what people would do. Let's say they have severe emphysema. They live at sea level San Francisco and even there they are severely short of breath; then they come up to an altitude of 4,500 feet and all of a sudden they can't breathe at all. We saw a lot of those cases over the years. They end up being hospitalized a couple of days to get them on their feet and get them back home.

Occasionally I get asked if I did house calls in my practice and I am pleased to say, "Yes." I made them from the time I entered practice in

1959 to the time I retired in 1993. I had several reasons for doing it. First, it was just the compassionate thing to do. A lot of times patients were quite sick and they needed attention. Maybe they were too sick or too feeble to get up and go to the emergency room. In that case, I would go see them, and then sometimes I did follow-up on other medical problems where they were still pretty sick after they left the hospital. Once they were home, I felt I needed to see them. They couldn't come into the office, so I would go see them. Second, I have always enjoyed house calls because I would see my patients in a home environment, which was a totally different experience from seeing them in the office with the formality of the doctor-patient relationship. Visiting with them on their own turf with their spouses, their children, or whatever, made for a different understanding of their needs and it made for a great relationship between my patients and me. They really appreciated that sort of thing and it became a natural function. I grew up with parents who did this. Again, that attitude was ingrained in me.

I am retired now but I still go see some of my patients. Sometimes they call me up and say, "Gee, I would like to see you," or something like that, so I go over on a social visit. I stay away from treating them, but sometimes they are not feeling well and haven't been able to contact their doctor. In a case like that I will get a hold of their doctor and tell him his patient should be seen today or tomorrow, or something like that. Their doctors usually appreciate that too.

In the first decade I was here, the 1960s, we had installed a small x-ray machine and did chest x-rays in the office. Both Fred Elliott and I utilized that modality, which was kind of unusual at that time, but we did it and it was very handy. We installed an electrocardiogram machine and did stair-step stress exams in our office too. Later we used treadmills for stress testing. Subsequently, we began using hospital facilities more and more for sophisticated testing. We used the radiology departments available in the hospitals all the time when we needed barium enema studies or other specialized testing for the gastrointestinal tract. This is long before we had Computerized Axial Tomography (CT) scans and the imaging equipment-technology that followed. Physicians had wonderful radiology support in both hospitals, not only for inpatients, but also for outpatients.

A Growing Practice

It's interesting that in the early 1960s before Medicare, my office visit charge was $5, which I reluctantly had to increase later to $7.50. My patients naturally objected to this increase too. When Medicare came in, things got a lot more complicated. Physicians didn't pay much attention to fees and such at that time. That part of the practice of medicine didn't appeal to most of us. I just did my work and let whatever happened in the way of collections take care of itself. Often a colleague would ask, "Well, how are your collections, are they eighty percent, ninety percent?" I never studied that. We were all making an adequate living and that seemed fair. A lot of times we just wrote off bad debts and I never sent anybody to collection; I never liked the concept of sending patients to collection agencies.

In 1970 Dr. Elliott and I moved our office to 975 Ryland Street over by Washoe Medical Center to be closer to the excellent radiology services there. Dr. Donald Day, another internist in Reno, had joined us in 1969 and we all stayed together until the mid-1970s when Fred started having heart problems. Fred ended up having major heart surgery in the late 1970s at Stanford. He had to get out of the practice of medicine, which had proven by this time to be too intense and demanding for him. He later ended up going to the VA Hospital as a staff member, which had even hours and was not too demanding, and he was able to finish his career that way.

Dr. Don Day and I stayed together in an association until I retired in 1993. We weren't necessarily in the same office space all the time, but we had a fine call arrangement. There were also a couple of other doctors involved with us at that time and our call schedules were complicated. A physician's free time is extremely limited and highly valued and a good working call arrangement has always been an essential part of medical practice. I had alternate weekends off. Then, when Dr. Day came along, we worked one weekend and we had two weekends off. Well, ultimately we got to a situation where we had four doctors taking call. This was a much more tolerable setup. Physician survival in this intense environment of medicine, I think, was due, in large part, to doctors organizing themselves in groups.

In my opinion, the large groups we now see associated do that primarily for the reason of providing respite time for physicians who have very intense practices. When they are on call, doctors get really involved and it often becomes a very stressful experience. They need frequent breaks from that intensity. The solo practitioner, the guy who took care of his own patients and took care of his own calls, is virtually non-existent in a community of this size. It may exist in very small communities, and I don't know how they work that out, but we see, for instance, large groups of cardiologists and pulmonary doctors in Reno joining forces because of the call requirements and that is very understandable to me. The drawback to this system is that the relationship between the doctor and patient is often confused.

The problem today is that a patient with a heart attack, for instance, can be admitted by one member of the cardiology group, and the doctor may not see that patient again for the entire time he is in the hospital. The patient will see a different doctor every day from that group who will manage everything as it comes up. From a medical standpoint, it is not a complicated thing to manage it, and they generally can do a good job at that, but the poor patient gets confused. He doesn't know who is his doctor. I have had physician friends, usually older doctors, admitted to a hospital for a major medical problem tell me, "John, I don't know who my heart doctor is."

Modern Medicine

Having many consultants and the patient not knowing their doctor is a part of modern medicine—an integral part of it, and unfortunately, it is not likely to change. It's a whole different breed of cat from the way medicine was practiced a generation ago. It also has something to do, I think, with the public's attitude towards physicians. The physician, a generation ago, was really pretty revered and held in the highest esteem. A lot of families were very happy about the idea of maybe one of their children going into medicine and considered that one of the top professions to go into. Patients today expect too much of their doctors; they expect to be cured at each encounter, and they can't deal with anything less than that. Medicine, and, unfortunately life, isn't necessarily that way.

There is a lot of information that is readily available to the patient. Formerly, it was available to the patient indirectly. A patient would be talking to his neighbor over the back fence. Then the patient would come into the office and say, "Mrs. Jones is taking this and she's got the same problems I have." Today, the patient has to be educated that Mrs. Jones does not have the same problem, and that it is totally different. The medication schedule is different because the health problems are not the same. After the situation has been explained, the patient eventually gets squared away. There is so much health information available, so much misinformation available, that patients are able to look on the Internet or see information on TV about a disease process or a great outcome. They then go to the doctor's office armed with all sorts of information they think is important. Some of it may be useful to the doctor, but a lot of it may just totally interfere with the patient's management because it is misguided and misunderstood. It becomes a complex problem for both the patient and the doctor.

Scientific knowledge and technology has progressed across the entire spectrum of the medical field. Radiology comes to mind because it became much more sophisticated with the development of arteriography, a procedure in which dye is injected into the blood stream and the circulation network can be evaluated directly and visually. This first became manifest in coronary arteriography, in which they are able to visualize the coronary circulation and locate blockages and judge how severe they were. This led to the development of coronary artery bypass surgery, which really became available in the late 1960s in university environs.

Another example, CT scans advanced our ability to diagnose disease processes. It is interesting that this technology became available in both our Reno hospitals almost immediately after it became available in the mid to late 1970s. Echocardiography utilizing ultrasound was next, in the late 1970s. Radiologists utilized it to look at gallbladders and abdominal disease processes and then to locate cardiac diseases. Both Washoe Medical Center and St. Mary's Hospital quickly acquired that technology and it has become extremely useful in diagnosing heart disease. This was a big advance. Magnetic resonance imaging arrived in Reno in the mid to late 1980s.

Although we looked at placing an echographic machine in our office, the costs would have been prohibitive. The expense was pretty tremendous and we couldn't justify it in a small practice. We utilized and capitalized on the availability of it at our hospitals and sent patients over there. Collectively, cardiologists have more economic power and they can bring this technology into their office and utilize it effectively there. We always tried to keep things simple in our office and I was able to retire in the early 1990s before I had to bring even a computer on board. I am grateful for that. But, that was then and if I'd stayed in practice another two years, I would have had to have a computer for the business aspect of things.

Fax machines came along and they sped up the process of getting patient's test results from the hospital almost instantaneously. We could have results in our hands immediately. That is great, and one can get information not only from a local community level, but also from other sources—universities, medical centers, and any place where important medical things are happening. I can't speak personally about the Internet, as I really don't know it all that well. I would suspect that the great majority of doctors probably utilize it today just the same way as the patients.

Doctors' time at the computer is going to do nothing but increase as time goes along. I saw something in the media recently where a doctor can now probably conduct an office visit from his home utilizing the computer, and robots now can assist surgeons in doing certain procedures. There seems to be no end to it. But, robots can't do it all and new technology can't do it all. The physician will always have to be there. As one surgeon at the Cleveland Clinic recently observed as he watched a robot-assisted procedure, "They sometimes get into trouble and they need us."

Dr. Frank E. Roberts

Early Life

I was born on March 13, 1928, and raised in Los Angeles where I graduated from high school in 1945 and attended the University of Southern California (USC). All my friends and family said I was destined to be a doctor, and that sounded like a good idea. Except for my godfather, who delivered me in Los Angeles, there were no other physicians in my immediate family. We were, however, surrounded by doctors where I grew up. One really nice physician I liked a lot lived next door and my brother and I played in his workshop with his kids. Another man who lived across the street was a former dean at the University of Southern California medical school. Although I knew nothing about medicine, I had continually been impressed with the physicians I had known and had been inspired by the few who had taken care of my medical needs over the years. All the doctors I had been associated with were fairly relaxed people, even though they had very busy practices. I guess they were well organized because I cannot remember one time when I had to wait a long time for my appointments.

Medical School and the U.S. Army

I entered the USC School of Medicine in 1949, after which I started a rotating internship program at the Los Angeles County General Hospital in 1953. Following my internship, I was accepted for an orthopedic residency at the New York Hospital for Bone and Joint Disease. I realized that by being an orthopedic surgeon one can easily lose sight of the whole patient if only treating an arm or a leg. In 1954 I interviewed for and was accepted in an internal medicine residency at the Los Angeles County Hospital; however, I chose the Mayo Clinic for my internal medicine training in Rochester, Minnesota, in October 1954. My ', Jean, and I had gotten married in July of 1954. We had our first child in November 1955, just before I was called into the army in December.

We were sent to Fort Sam Houston in San Antonio, Texas, and I learned how to march and do all that military stuff before being transferred to Camp Irwin, a training facility in Barstow, California. We were there until December 1957, and then we returned to Rochester to finish my internal medicine residency. The time in Barstow was just delightful. It was January when we returned to the Mayo Clinic and it was cold and icy. Jean was expecting our second child, Kathy, who was born in January 1958.

During my duty in the army, we spent some time driving all over California looking for cities and towns to start my practice. We eliminated lots of places, and the idea of settling in Reno became more and more appealing as time went by. I knew Carroll Ogren, administrator at Washoe County Hospital, Jack Streeter, a former District Attorney, and several builders in Reno.

Internal Medicine in Reno (Roberts)

Move to Reno

In January 1960 we moved to Reno, rented a place, and immediately began building a house. Our twins were born in March 1961. I opened a solo practice in an office on the corner of California and Arlington Avenues and began building my practice. There were some very nice doctors in that building. Dr. Ernie Mack, a neurosurgeon, was on one side, while Dr. Les Gould, a psychiatrist, was my other neighbor.[2] Down the hall there were Drs. John Ervin, Gilbert Lenz, Mortimer Falk, and John Sande.[3] Dr. Nick Landis, another internist, was doing some subspecialty work in oncology and he was the first oncologist in town.[4] Also in that building were Sam Zive, a physical therapist, and Radiologist Harry Gilbert who had an office in the basement. A pediatric group composed of Drs. John Palmer, John Scott, Emanuel Berger, and William Pasutti were also tenants in the building.

At that time, there were only about ten or so internal medicine specialists in town, so my days went by very quickly; there was plenty of work. I got to do a lot of emergency room work since we didn't have any full-time ER doctors in town, and I made a lot of house, hotel, and motel visits. People would call and say they had somebody really drunk in their motel room, urging me to give something to quiet them down. I became busy right from the start, and I can remember getting calls from the Holiday Hotel asking me to come in to take care of someone. I would be paid $20 for that "hotel" call when my office visits would be between $5 and $7.50. House calls were wonderful and I enjoyed them a lot. During those visits, I got to know families very well.

Internists in Reno

When I first came to town, there were five internists covering for each other on weekends and evenings: Drs. Dave Roberts, Bob Myles, Claude Belcourt, sometimes John Davis, and Fred Elliott. Dr. Claude Belcourt joined me later when he left his associate, Dr. Horace Taylor.[5] In 1965, we moved to a new office at 890 Mill Street, which had just been built, but was not completely finished. In 1968 Dr. David Johnson joined Dr. Belcourt and me. We all made rounds at the hospital together on Mondays and Fridays. Patients got to know all of us pretty well. We used to have the best and the most lively exchanges over diagnoses. During the week, we took care of our own patients and I think this call and rounds-sharing was unique—even today I think it would be considered unique. The patients really appreciated it.

We were managing our time quite well and our families benefited greatly. It worked well for us; if I was away and one of my patients needed to be seen, he came in and would have already met the doctor taking my call. Obstetricians/gynecologists do that a lot. They cycle the doctors through who will be on-call when their patients are most likely to deliver.

In the beginning I knew all of the doctors in town. I don't think there were any physicians I didn't know after I was in Reno a couple of years. I frequently consulted with them or visited with them at meetings, but as the society got bigger, the attendance at the meetings got worse. I once went to a meeting in Hawaii, which has a huge medical community, and there were only twelve people there. In the early and mid-1960s, when we had meetings in Reno, almost every doctor in town would be there because, for one, it was a social thing, and two, it was important because so much was going on at that time. They were all my good friends and I always looked forward to seeing them.

Economics of Practice

The economics of medicine began to change as time went by. I had to increase my fees because people had stopped coming. This seemed to be the reverse of what usually happens in business. My associate, Dr. Claude Belcourt, and I called in an accountant, LeRoy Bergstrom, to help sort things out. He told us what was going on and advised us to raise our fees. After we did that, we became busier than we had ever been. That was amazing and didn't make any sense. We began seeing more patients. A $20 bottle of wine must be better than a $10 bottle of wine, even though they both cost $5 to make.

I had trained at the Mayo Clinic in Rochester and there were a lot more consultative services available to me there than when I first came to Reno. Back at Mayo there were always numerous subspecialists standing by. If I had a patient with an ulcer problem or a blood pressure problem, I could always get a consultant to see my patient. In Reno, in the early days we didn't have that luxury—we had to be our own consultant. We did have an excellent laboratory available and there were good radiologists and outstanding surgeons in the basic specialties. I don't recall much out-of-area referral going on except in areas such as heart surgery. There were some challenging patients and I recall one with ulcerative colitis that we tried everything that we knew to do before referring the patient out. Patients didn't really mind going out-of-state for medical care that was not available here. For example, it was not a big trip for patients to go over to Sacramento to have heart-valve surgery performed.

At that time subspecialists weren't available in every nook and cranny of most states. They pretty much stayed in the areas around teaching institutions, but that began to change in the late 1960s and 1970s. I never felt short-changed. Technology found in the major teaching centers got better and better and began to hit Reno, and I think we were very much up-to-date except for a very few items. I think the arrival of Computerized Axial Tomography (CT) scans, Magnetic Resonance Imaging (MRI), and things of that sort weren't really behind other areas in general.

Explosion of Medical Technology

There was an explosion in medical technology in the mid-1970s and it is continuing today. In medicine it is critically important for us to know what we don't know, and I think that is what we practice on a daily basis. We quickly become familiar with what we don't know. That is one of the most frustrating parts about managed care—we know a patient needs to be seen by a physician with special training and we're prevented from referring. I had trouble with this, but I saw it coming before I retired. I did most of my practice at Washoe Medical Center just because it was a busier hospital and had an emergency room, which Saint Mary's didn't have until sometime later. I picked up a lot of patients because I took frequent call in the ER, so my time was better spent there. Washoe administration was generally considered to be a very tight ship. Carroll Ogren, the hospital administrator, and the head nurse, Maida Pringle, would make rounds on all patients everyday. Administration did the same at Saint Mary's Hospital; Sister Seraphine would visit each patient every day. I can't imagine that being done today. It kind of reminds me of going to a restaurant and having the maitre'd come over and asking, "How are you?"

When I came to town in 1960, the major part of the hospital was the old brick building on the corner of Kirman and Mill Streets, and I am not quite sure when it was built, probably around the turn of the century, I would guess. [It was built in 1906.] After an early beginning, Washoe proceeded to grow farther out to the east and later the Pringle Building was built. Carroll Ogren saw to it that every bit of construction was first class and no corners were cut. Good design work and engineering went into making it a pleasant place to work.

There used to be a coffee room right by the old surgical suite at Washoe, and we would all go there and have coffee, or a donut, or whatever was around. So all of these people would be there and I talked to them and was brought up to speed on the medical and political issues of the day. There would be times, too, when I would need a surgical consultation, which I could set up at that time. Then as the hospital got bigger, the coffee room became an office and it was moved close to surgery down in the basement. It became hard to get to and the social thing seemed to disappear. People now are just going, going all the time.

Possibly the first publicly visible technological advance at the hospital was the arrival of the helicopter with a landing pad located across the street from Pickett Park.[6] There were many doctors who thought the helicopter was kind of silly and more than a little bit dangerous. Those things do crash. But I think they came to realize that it provided a valuable service to outlying areas, as the speed of retrieval is quite important in auto accidents and such. Some even began to think of the helicopter as a prestigious thing for the medical center even though it was shared with Saint Mary's Hospital.

With every technological advance such as CT, MRI, and the helicopter, there is an increase in the costs of healthcare and the same goes for advances in pharmaceuticals and medical procedures. One pays for what one gets. I always paid close attention to the costs of medicines I prescribed and lab tests I ordered. For example, it might be considerably cheaper to order a complete chemistry panel rather than a few specific tests. My patients always appreciated this. The new medicines that have come out during my career have been impressive and have made things better for patients, as many of the new drugs have fewer side-effects, last longer, and generally are more effective than the ones they replace. The internet also has been a big help with researching these newer drugs and can be a valuable aid in prescribing, and computers have certainly eased the burden of patients billing. The computer does it all and at the end of the day, paper work is current.

I never liked the idea of members of a physician's staff practicing medicine. I think it is wrong. The few times a patient sees me in a year warrants my attention, not that of a nurse or a physician's assistant. I just don't like taking care of patients unless I am personally involved.

In looking back over my years in medicine I think the most

important advances have been in the development of new pharmaceuticals such as antihypertensives, antibiotics, and ulcer medications. I also think that the development and contributions made by subspecialties within internal medicine, along with laboratory and x-ray advances, have been immensely important.

Notes
[1] Dr. Frederick Elliott as born in Pennsylvania in 1914 and licensed in Nevada in 1948.

[2] Dr. Leslie Gould was born in California in 1921 and licensed in Nevada in 1956.

[3] Dr. Mortimer Falk was born in NY in 1919 and licensed in Nevada in 1951.Dr. Gilbert Lenz, a general surgeon, was born in Wisconsin in 1919 and licensed in Nevada in 1955.Dr. John Sande graduated from the Univ. of Minn. in 1950 and was licensed in Nevada in 1958.

[4] Dr. Nick Landis was born in Pennsylvania in 1910 and licensed in Nevada in 1946.

[5] Dr. Horace Taylor was born in Massachusetts in 1921 and licensed in Nevada in 1953,

[6] Bill Lear provided the first helicopter in 1970s, but it was discontinued because it was too expensive. Its value was demonstrated in Vietnam, and it came to Reno in 1978.

6: Dr. Adolf Rosenauer, Neurosurgery

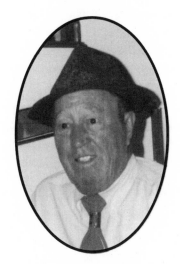

Dr. Adolf Rosenauer

Early Life

I was born in Linz, Austria on September 20, 1922. Linz, which means the place in a river that can be forded, is an ancient town dating back before the time of the Romans. It is Celtic in origin and the name appears in many places in the Alps.

Austria is a small country, which measures only about one-third the size of Nevada with a population of barely seven million people. Today over one-third of Austrians live in Vienna, the capitol city. There are over 260 million people living in the u.s....imagine if over eighty-six million of us lived in Washington, D.C.

My father owned and operated a grocery store that had been in the Rosenauer family for two generations. He had the equivalent of a bachelor's degree and had served in ww i. He always had an interest in studying economics at the university, but those studies were permanently interrupted when his father suddenly died and he had to take over operation of the grocery store.

I began school when I was six years old and finished what might be called high school in 1940. I can remember having to recite the names of all the states in the u.s. There were only forty-eight at that time. We attended school five and a half days a week and a lot of time was spent going back and forth to school, so in order to shorten this time and make it economical, my father allowed me to buy an old bicycle. I say allowed because I had to earn the money to buy it, and I did that by tutoring other students. The tutoring business wasn't all that difficult for me because most of the time I was first in my class. That bicycle cut the travel time down considerably. I was as active as I could be in sports like soccer and ice hockey, but actually there was little time for that. Physics, chemistry, mathematics, history, and geography were my first interests, and I benefited from that early concentration on academics.

Early in my studies I had decided to be a doctor. My mother was an army nurse in the First World War and my uncle was a Vienna-trained surgeon. In a way, that decision was made rather quickly because of the economics of the times; there wasn't much time to ponder a career.

I knew that medical school would be a long hard pull. In Austria it was a five-year, ten-semester course of study and courses were graded with eighteen examinations over those years. Theoretically it was possible to reduce that somewhat if one crammed, but it usually took eleven semesters because some courses required more intensive study than others.

The German Army

Before I could concentrate on my studies, I had to go into the military. Men had to serve two years in the army, but if we enlisted voluntarily before being drafted, that service was reduced to one year; most of the young men did just that. I volunteered at seventeen. Years later I was asked which side I fought for during the war and I replied, "I fought against Stalin."

The first six months of military service was composed of a period called the "CCC," which was a "pick and shovel" for everyone regardless of education or background.

When my year's service was over, I entered the University of Innsbruck in what was called an "inscribed status." After three months, I was called back into service because the war was still in full swing and I had only been in school three months. I asked my professor if I could somehow get credit for the full semester. He challenged me to get the signatures of all of my professors in order to get full credit. I quickly and excitedly got those signatures, and this proved to be very important later on.

I was sent to Munich and became trained as a radioman. Later the big shots found out they did not have enough doctors, so they rounded up all the medical students, and we were transferred over to the medical corps. I wasn't quite through with the six weeks of retraining when, in 1941, I was transferred to Minsk, the capital of White Russia.

It was a lousy war, I mean really lousy. Every soldier I ever knew had lice, not just a few of them, but thousands. De-lousing was not very effective and chloromycetin, which held out to be somewhat promising, did not come along until later. At that time lice were everywhere and, as a result of this infestation, I contracted typhus in 1942 and became quite ill. It turned out to be the major killer in German concentration camps. As there was no treatment, a fifty- percent fatality rate was not unusual.

When I got out of the hospital after being treated for typhus, I couldn't walk very far, but at least I was upright again. I wasn't certain what my job was going to be in the medical corps, but I was glad I had the medical student designation. Some of us were being sent back to the university for more study and once we had that one semester under our belts, we were sent to a combat unit. This was a little different for me because the unit I was assigned to was destroyed, so I got sent back to Munich and ultimately to Innsbruck for more study. This tour of duty continued for two years before I was shipped out again, this time to Yugoslavia.

I was assigned to an army field hospital and things were very quiet for quite a spell; there was no artillery and no shooting. Things changed when the British Air Force came and bombed the city repeatedly, and I remember one time they hit the gypsy quarters and that was a blood-bath. Body parts were flying everywhere. One wonders why the British bombed hospitals with the Red Cross all over them, but I suspect they were flying so high they could not see the crosses.

When we were ready to leave the area, railroad control officers bumped us off the train. That particular train was supposed to take us out of the combat zone. The train we finally boarded the next day soon passed the train we were originally to take. The tracks were destroyed and everyone on that train was dead.

I made it home to Linz for Christmas that year and was immediately reassigned to Italy. I sort of had two assignment choices at that time: Krakow, Poland or Adria, a small town near Venice. Not much of a problem choosing on that one.

Not long after I got to Italy we were told the war was over and to go home the best way we could. In May 1945, I made my way on foot across the Alps toward Linz and home.

The situation was sad at home. While my mother was alive, my brother had died, and it took my father over six months to get back to Linz. The grocery store was still there and was pretty much cleaned out.

Medical Education

I was still considered a medical student at that time, so I went to the hospital in Linz, which belonged to the Order of the Brothers of Charity.

At one time my Uncle Fritz was a doctor there and when the hospital was taken over by the Germans, Uncle Fritz was made chief surgeon. I was impressed with the fact that he was part of the group that officially surrendered Linz to the American army. Had they not done that, the town was to be bombed completely as it was definitely marked for destruction.

After the surrender of Linz, an American doctor named Zwalsch was assigned to run the hospital, which was designated to handle prisoners of war, and he approached Uncle Fritz saying, "I can't run this hospital. I don't know how to do that. Let's make an agreement. You tell me what has to be done and I will sign the orders." And so the two of them worked together just perfectly until the Brothers of Charity returned and the hospital was handed back over to them. When his tour of duty was over, Dr. Zwalsch returned to his practice in Idaho, but came back frequently to visit my uncle.

I returned to the University of Innsbruck and completed my medical degree in 1947, and for a year or two afterwards, I was assistant professor of anatomy at Innsbruck. Then I left and went to my Uncle Fritz's hospital in Linz because I was quite interested in some microscopic studies on the sympathetic nervous system and Uncle Fritz did a lot of sympathectomies. So I got specimens fresh from patients and at night I would do microscopic studies in a laboratory I set up in Uncle Fritz's apartment.

During that time I met a physician named Joe Evans, a professor of neurosurgery at the University of Cincinnati and also a member of the World Health Commission. He invited me to come to Cincinnati to replace a research assistant who, in Joe's eyes, was not as critical as he should be in his microscopic anatomy studies. It took a while, but I eventually accepted the assignment and traveled to Ohio, courtesy of the Rockefeller Foundation.

The Move to the United States
The Rockefeller Foundation arranged for me to have a visitor's visa to the United States and a stipend of two hundred dollars per month; that was back in 1951 and as I was single at the time, this income seemed to be quite satisfactory to me.

At the university, I was required to continue my studies and enrolled in numerous prescribed courses, which led to my taking and passing the examination for a Master of Science degree. One of the questions the examiner asked me on American literature was, "Have you ever heard of a writer with the name of Henry Wadsworth Longfellow?" Was it a coincidence that I had just finished reading Hiawatha? That clinched it. I was awarded the M.S. degree.

Dr. Evans asked me to take over the job as chief resident in the neurosurgery program at the hospital as the current man had gotten an abscessed tooth and became quite ill. I got full credit for the year I spent there. The Rockefeller Foundation extended my agreement for another year and even granted me the opportunity to return to Austria with paid passage.

At that time, I had learned there was a professor of neuropsychiatry and neurosurgery at Innsbruck who, although a very learned man, was, in a word, impossible to get along with. He was head of the department where I would be working if I were to return to Austria, and, I must say, I had second thoughts about returning. This professor, a man named Hubert Urban, had come to Innsbruck in 1937 and had been denied privileges to teach at the university. He then left, spent four years teaching in Brazil, London, San Francisco, and Norway, and returned to Austria. With his new credentials and contacts, he convinced administration at Innsbruck to accept him and they did. I suspect they must have said, "We will have to take this man, but God help us!" Once there, nobody could work with this fellow; several physicians left the university.

I went to the Rockefeller Foundation in New York and notified them I would not be able to work in Innsbruck with this Dr. Urban, and they said they would investigate the matter. Although not going back to Austria was a big disappointment for me, I was satisfied with my lot to continue my studies and training at Cincinnati.

It wasn't long before Dr. Evans relocated to the University of Chicago. I went with him and spent a year there as an instructor in neurosurgery. I believe the year was 1954. As I was finishing up my residency training (I even spent one more year as instructor and chief resident at the Billings hospital), I had lots of people approach me to relocate to their states and their facilities, but state licensure requirements varied so much. For example, in some states they required another year of training in addition to what I had already finished.

The Move to Nevada

It seemed that Nevada had the most reasonable requirements for licensure and that interested me quite a lot. Dr. Ernest Wood Mack of Reno had come to the University of Chicago and inquired of Professor Joe Evans if he knew of anyone who could help him in his practice in Nevada.[1] Of course, I came highly recommended by Dr. Evans and that is how I wound up in Reno in 1957.

The year previous to coming to Reno, I took a trip to Europe and it was there I married Eva Moore from Portland whom I had met on the boat trip over. We had our first child, Patricia, in Chicago; then relocated to Reno. We have been married forty-six years and successfully raised Patricia, Michael, and Kathleen.

Neurosurgery in Reno

Naturalization and Exam for Licensure

When I got to Reno, it came time for me to become a naturalized u.s. citizen and a whole new process opened up. I formerly had made application for naturalization, but the laws were changed and all the "first" papers I had previously filed had to be re-done. In addition, it was an election year and the naturalization process was put on hold during that period because of the potential for voting irregularities. For example, I had heard that a well-known Nevada u.s. Senator, Pat McCarran, was suspected of bringing in trainloads of Mexicans on election day when he first ran for congress. There was very little doubt that he did this; they voted for him and then he sent them home the next day. It was evident then that there were far more votes cast that day for the senator than there were citizens in Nevada so a law was enacted to put naturalizations on hold during elections.

I had to wait a year to become a citizen. Also, I had to go before the Nevada State Board of Medical Examiners under the direction of Dr. Kenneth Maclean.[2] He told me that he knew all about my training and that he knew who I was and knew of my performance at the University of Cincinnati and the University of Chicago. He passed me and I got a license to practice medicine. However, about a week later he told me he needed to get my license back. He said he couldn't explain it now, but he would tell me later. He also asked me whether I could write a Nevada state medical exam, which I told him, "Yes, any time you say so," after all, I had been an academic teacher for years. In due time I was asked to write the basic science, as well as the clinical science exams and so I became one of the few colleagues who actually wrote a Nevada state medical examination. The Board of Medical Examiners gave me the license (actually the "second one") to practice medicine in Nevada shortly afterwards.

Shortly after I completed my licensure exam, a colleague from the Veterans Hospital asked me what I had to do to be issued a license. I told him that I simply passed a Nevada state medical exam. Then I found out that things were a little more complicated. The colleague who asked me was a certain Dr. Frommer. He was a Jewish refugee from Vienna from the late 1930s, and when he arrived in New York City, he was given a license to practice medicine. Many years later when the Veterans Administration inquired about his graduation from the University of Vienna, they were told there never was a graduate by that name. Later, Dr. Maclean told me that this was the reason he wanted me to pass this Nevada State medical exam.

Until I became a citizen, I was employed at the Washoe County Hospital as the area's first electro-encephalographer, and things went quite smoothly. With that employment and my working with Dr. Bill Mack, I was in charge of practically all neurosurgery of indigent patients in Washoe County.

Reno Neurosurgeons

When I began my practice in Reno, Dr. Mack had been here since 1946 and had gained a national reputation for his work. He was joined later by Dr. Charles Fleming, and then I came along and it stayed that way for several years until other neurosurgeons came.[3] Sometime later a number of colleagues, Drs. Bob Morelli, Lou Levy, Bill Dawson, and Joe Walker came to town. Dr. Alan Mischler came and he had a short and unsettling practice. He lost all hospital privileges, and eventually lost his license to practice medicine in Nevada.

At that time there were fewer than four hundred neurosurgeons in the entire country and they all knew each other quite well. Just a few years later there were over a thousand and that is the way the specialty of neurosurgery has grown over the years.

State-of-the-Art Neurosurgery

The state of the art in Reno in the field of neurosurgery was excellent when I came here. Dr. Mack had a fine reputation, as did Dr. Chuck Fleming, and imaging equipment at both hospitals was quite good. I brought the percutaneous angiogram procedure to the area: a procedure whereby the doctor sticks a needle into the carotid artery to do a vascular study. Before this arrived on the scene, the neurosurgeon would do an invasive procedure and open the patient's neck and insert the catheter into the artery. Neurodiagnostic studies of the brain using contrast media were in their infancy, and we learned that contrast media used in x-rays of the brain were often very toxic, but contrast media was improved over the years.

In the early days we did a procedure to immobilize neck and spinal cord-injured patients. We put the patient in a cast that went down to the hipbone with a stiff neck brace and an immobilizing head ring so the patient was prevented from moving. This was then replaced by the halo brace with its head screws. Later on technology advanced to where, through improved imaging, we could localize the injury quite well and have more treatment options. Some neurosurgeons began studying neuroradiology, which requires an additional three years in radiology residency programs.

In vogue at the time were procedures labeled "lobotomies" and "lobectomies," and these were commonly called patient "tranquilizers." They were fairly destructive and physicians who repeatedly performed them were not thought of very highly. However, it was understood that certain personality features associated with rabid, angry, volatile, and destructive behaviors disappeared or were greatly reduced if the frontal lobe was de-activated; that was the chief benefit of those procedures. I think over my early career I had done relatively very few of them and then only in extreme circumstances.

Those procedures fell into disfavor over the years, as effective tranquilizing and much less toxic medications began appearing on the scene. In the early days, however, there was certain hesitancy in doing lobotomies as they destroyed parts of the brain. We would look for all kinds of alternatives to get away from doing them.

Then specific medications to combat brain tumors came along. We found that some tumors were highly sensitive to drugs. We were able to localize them and facilitate their removal with as little bleeding as possible. With the advent of Computerized Axial Tomography (CAT), Magnetic Resonance Imaging (MRI), and later Positron Emission Tomography (PET) machines, a whole new world opened up to neurosurgeons in Reno and across the nation. Washoe Medical Center always kept up with these technologically advanced, but very expensive, pieces of equipment.

There is much talk about Alzheimer's disease (AD). I have a slightly different opinion about this diagnosis than many neurosurgeons. Dr. Alzheimer described this condition in his papers written in 1890, and many doctors today label patients with "dementia" as "Alzheimer's disease." I have a hunch that former President Ronald Reagan's condition was termed Alzheimer's disease in order not to say he had senile dementia and his personal friends and staff knew this. In my experience, most cases of AD I have seen over the years progressed quite rapidly, as senile dementia does not. I once had a patient who went from being perfectly normal to a babbling idiot. He had to be tied to a table in just a matter of months—perhaps one year. Now, that's Alzheimer's, not this matter of being occasionally forgetful.

There have been many advances in my field over the years and this would make it seem that future neurosurgeons might not have to spend one third of their lives in the hospital, but that is the way it has been for many of us. One time I logged twenty-three straight nights in the hospital, and that really grinds a man down. Toward the end of my career, I gradually reduced my surgeries, which led to a slowing of my office practice and eventually to my doing what I call bureaucratic work, like physical examinations, lawyer work, and chart reviews. Before that, however, I did considerable work for the health plans and HMOs that began moving in, but this was a gradual process and I cannot say all my experiences with those plans were good.

The medical liability insurance crisis hit in the early 1970s and continued up until my retirement. I remember going with Ken Maclean to Yerington, Nevada, once to consult with Dr. Mary Fulstone, the longtime family doctor there.[4] We were always glad to travel to that small rural town because Dr. Mary was a very bright rural doctor who knew exactly when to call for assistance. Dr. Maclean asked her if she was feeling the strain of the costs of medical malpractice insurance and she asked, "What is that?" Dr. Mary never had the need for that insurance because of her relationships with her patients.

I see steady progress being made in the field of neurosurgery in the years ahead. Remarkable progress has already been made in treating aneurysms of the brain, a dreaded thing. The advent of arteriography and the steady decrease in the toxicity of the substances used has been such a big advance in helping surgeons locate tumors faster and with greater safety. New radiological advances with new dyes being used have reduced the need for craniotomies, but I must say that radiologic treatment of deep-seated brain tumors has made little progress in recent years. On the other hand, new chemotherapeutic agents have made remarkable strides.

Surgical techniques for managing tumors and aneurysms have also advanced. Patients have benefited enormously from the use of smaller instruments, the increase in the use of microscopes, and the use of equipment with coaxial light.

I do think all the research with DNA molecules, gene mapping, and splicing, may cause us to lose more than we hope to gain. The central nervous system (CNS) has continually been finicky about scientists' attempts at promoting cell regeneration. Yes, we can continually assist the CNS in searching out new nerve pathways, new rewiring, but that is about all there is at present. Successful stem cell transplantation and CNS cell regrowth is far in the future.

I do not wish to sound too negative for not holding out much hope for dramatic advances in the field of neurosurgery in the immediate future. I still do my best to keep up with the literature in my field, but I do not see much on the horizon.

Eva and I have been very happy in Reno all these years and feel we have made a contribution to our community and to the state. We have seen Reno grow, perhaps too much, but through it all we have enjoyed wonderful friends and a bright medical community. We are looking forward to retirement years—to enjoy our children and grandchildren, our farm animals, and our yearly trips back to Europe.

Notes

[1] Dr. Ernest "Bill" Mack was born in Nevada in 1913 and licensed in Nevada after World War II.

[2] Dr. Kenneth Maclean was born in Nevada in 1914 and licensed in Nevada in 1945.

[3] Dr. Charles Fleming was born in Nevada in 1925 and licensed in Nevada in 1956.

[4] Dr. Mary Fulstone was born in Nevada in 1892 and licensed in Nevada in 1920.

7: Dr. Ronald Avery, Obstetrics and Gynecology

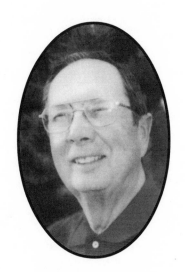

Dr. Ronald Avery

Education

I was born October 3, 1936, in Lake Village, Arkansas, a small town in the Mississippi river delta on the border of Louisiana and Mississippi. Lake Village is largely a farming community. When I was growing up, the population was around fifteen hundred, and it hasn't changed much over the years. The county has Arkansas's largest natural lake, Lake Chicot, an ox bow lake formed when the Mississippi River changed its course.

I wanted to be a doctor from an early age and ran around with two friends whose fathers were physicians. We spent a lot of time hanging out at the local hospital and it seemed natural that I would be a doctor someday. My father worked for the post office and my mother was a bank teller, so I knew that I would have to work to supplement my college and medical school education. Dr. Burge, my friend's father, was an inspiration to me and always encouraged me to follow my dream.

There were thirty-four people in my high school graduating class and three of us became physicians. One is a general surgeon who returned to Lake Village to practice with his father; another is a psychiatrist in San Francisco.

I attended Arkansas A & M College in Monticello, Arkansas, which is now an extension of the University of Arkansas. That first year was tough! I spent a total of six hundred dollars for room, board, books, and miscellaneous. This was made possible only by eating most of my meals in my room. My roommate and I had a hotplate, and we would use it nearly every night—a can of beans for dinner one night, and a can of corn the next. I would hitchhike sixty miles back home to Lake Village once in a while and take my laundry for my mother to clean. The few pennies saved on laundry meant an occasional decent meal for me.

I received my Bachelor's of Science in Chemistry from Arkansas A & M, and I was accepted at the University of Arkansas School of Medicine in Little Rock. Arkansas was regarded as a very good medical school. I received an excellent education: one that prepared me for later studies and my career. Our class started with one hundred students and graduated seventy-four. Arkansas traditionally eliminated twenty-five percent. Acceptance to medical school did not automatically mean that one would graduate. Receiving my M.D. was a lifelong dream come true.

Internship

After medical school, I did a rotating internship at Confederate Memorial Medical Center in Shreveport, Louisiana. Confederate Memorial was an excellent training facility and the experience was invaluable. There were forty interns and we staffed the various hospital services thirty-six hours on duty and twelve hours off. Rotating internship has all but disappeared. The new doctor today goes directly from medical school into a specialty residency program. Even general practice requires a three-year residency after medical school.

My wife, Judy, and I were married in June of 1962, just a few weeks after I completed medical school. Judy graduated the same year from St. Olaf College in Northfield, Minnesota, with a Bachelor's of Science in Nursing. We met at Anoka State Mental Hospital in Anoka, Minnesota, in the summer of 1960 when Judy was going through her psychiatric rotation and I was doing an externship.

U.S. Air Force

The Vietnam War was heating up about this time and every able-bodied man had to go into the service. After my internship, I had the option of either volunteering and going into the military as a general medical officer with the rank of captain or being drafted and serving my country in the army as a private. As this was not a difficult choice, I volunteered for the air force and boldly applied for a slot in California. I instead was sent to Greenville, Mississippi. The military must have thought they were pulling a real fast one on me—thinking that a tour of duty there would be just awful, but Greenville was a nice place and only twenty miles from home.

I first went to Montgomery, Alabama, for three weeks of basic training to learn to salute, march, and fire a rifle. During this time, orders were being re-written and many of my colleagues on base were being sent to Vietnam. I figured it was off to "Nam" for me as well, but my orders remained unchanged and I stayed at Greenville.

The Air Force Base at Greenville was small and the hospital was staffed with six brand new general medical officers and one military physician administrator. Each general medical officer had to "mini" specialize. One doctor had a year of an internal medicine residency and became the base internist. Another doctor with a year of general surgery training became the surgeon. I was sent off for a crash course in radiology and became the base radiologist. I liked radiology and briefly considered it for a specialty, but soon realized that I was a "people person" and that radiology would not be a good choice for me. During my tour at Greenville, I spent time with some of the local obstetricians and decided the specialty that encompassed most of my interests (general practice, internal medicine, surgery, and psychiatry) was obstetrics and gynecology. I have, over the years, thoroughly enjoyed my patients and practice, and have never regretted my choice.

My military tour of duty was for two years, but for reasons unexplained, it was decided that the base would be shut down after I has been there only eighteen months. I was given the choice of extending my military service for another year or taking an early discharge. Again, the choice was not difficult, and due to a vacancy in the program, I was able to immediately enter an obstetrics and gynecology residency at the University of Arkansas Medical Center in Little Rock.

Residency

I was fortunate to train under Dr. Willis Brown, a well-known obstetrician/gynecologist. He was a brilliant clinician and practitioner and had the honor to be president of the American College of Obstetricians and Gynecologists in 1968. He would have become a specialist in gynecologic oncology had there been such a subspecialty back then. The university medical center was both a research and teaching hospital. Indigents who needed special care were treated and it was the referral hospital for the whole state of Arkansas.

Residency was labor-intensive and poorly reimbursed. I made $275 per month that first year. Dr. Brown's residency was tough, but those who finished the program were well trained and experienced. First year residents had to work thirty-six hours on and twelve hours off the entire year. The pace lessened somewhat the second year. The hours were still long, but occasionally one could moonlight at one of the local emergency rooms to make a little extra money. Judy got a job teaching pediatric nursing at St. Vincent's Hospital in Little Rock. Her job paid the bills and kept us going for the next two and a half lean years.

The third year was even better. Residents had to spend a lot of time in the ob/gyn indigent clinics. Three months were spent on the gynecologic pathology service, and one month doing general anesthesia in the operating room. Interestingly, in the early 1960s, obstetrical and gynecologic residency programs across the nation were commonly three-year programs, but at Arkansas, it was a full four years.

My fourth year as chief resident (I was now making $500 per month) was divided between obstetrics, general gynecology, and gynecologic oncology.

We did numerous gynecologic vaginal and abdominal surgeries, and most of our own urological procedures. On obstetrics, we took care of the complicated obstetrical problems, deliveries, and c-sections. On gynecologic oncology, we performed various radical procedures, and did our own radiation dosage calculations and implants. This last year honed our skills and gave us the added knowledge, practice, and confidence with which to enter the private sector.

Obstetrics and Gynecology in Reno

Move to Reno

My coming to Reno was purely accidental. I was a southern boy and it was understood that I would practice somewhere in the South. During my last year of residency, Judy and I looked at several potential practice locations, but we were not excited by any of them. Then my chief got a call from Dr. Bill Bynum, a Reno obstetrician/gynecologist. He and his colleague, Dr. Robert Stewart, were looking for a graduating resident to come into their practice. Their senior partner, Dr. Silas Ross, had recently died. I flew to Reno without my wife to look things over.[1] Reno was a very nice, small town in 1968. There were three to four high-rise buildings (the Mapes, First National Bank, Arlington Towers, and the apartment towers across the river), two hospitals, and only about one hundred thousand people in the Reno/Sparks metropolitan area. Lake Tahoe was beautiful, and San Francisco and the entire Northwest were readily accessible. We had two children at that time. Our daughter, Suzanne, was born in 1964 during our military tour of duty in Greenville, Mississippi. Our son, Ron III, was born during my year as chief resident in 1967 in Little Rock. Judy was eager to move West and trusting my impressions we decided to move to Reno. We came and stayed, and in 1971, we had our third child, Robert, a native Nevadan.

Reno Obstetricians

The medical community was small, under one hundred physicians, when I arrived in Reno. There were twelve or thirteen obstetricians and gynecologists included in that number. Most of them were in solo practice, but there were a few groups. Dr. Clare Wolfe, Tom Mullis, and Paul Wigg were solo, but were not delivering babies.[2] Drs. Jack Stapleton and George Furman were by themselves. Everyone knew everybody, and the physicians were all easy to work with.

I stayed with Drs. Stewart and Bynum for about ten months. I left their group to do solo practice, but was instead persuaded by Dr. Jack Stapleton to join him. We were together until he quit obstetrics, and I went on my own in 1975.

My practice grew very rapidly and I had more than I could do after a very short time. After 1970, we needed to limit the number of new patients we could accept. I was working a hundred hours a week. Several of the years that Jack and I were together, we were averaging sixty deliveries a month, each one of us doing no fewer than four or five major surgeries a week, plus seeing fifty patients a day in the office.

Gynecologic Pathology in Reno

There was a lot of gynecologic pathology for a community of Reno's size back then. In those early years, there was a fair amount of cervical cancer. This type of cancer is rarely seen today due to the increased awareness and acceptance of Pap smear testing. Obstetrics was challenging as well. We did not have fetal monitors, fetal stress testing equipment, or ultrasound. Technical advances have greatly improved fetal outcome, maternal health, and well being.

Advances in Obstetrics and Gynecology

It is really hard to say what would be the greatest single technological improvement in my specialty over the past thirty years. There have been so many advancements. The ultrasound was of tremendous benefit to obstetrics. It contributed to the diagnosis of congenital abnormalities and multiple pregnancies, and helped in establishing infant size and pregnancy dating. Prenatal health was more easily monitored, and early detection and treatment in pregnancy led to reduced infant morbidity and mortality. As for gynecology, the laparoscope advanced surgical technique to a high degree. Its use cut down on pain, reduced the size of incisions, shortened the hospital stay, and made patient recovery better and faster. The culposcope and LEEP machine were also important new technologies. Gynecologists could now diagnose and treat precancerous lesions and other abnormalities of the cervix in the office, thereby eliminating some hospital admissions.

Advances and improvements in pharmaceuticals have also been significant over the course of my career. Medicines have become better and new antibiotics have saved countless patients who previously may have died from their infections.

Numerous studies have been done regarding hormone replacement therapy, and we now test to see if women are in the menopause. There are new and different types of hormone replacement medication as well as alternative methods of treatment to alleviate the symptoms and adverse effects of menopause and aging.

There are now numerous tests to identify, treat, and follow-up different types of cancers. There are mammography and ultrasound to identify breast cancer and chemical markers to follow those patients being treated. There are many new improvements in chemotherapeutic agents and radiation techniques. There are new tests for ovarian cancer, but these are not yet as sensitive or as absolute to diagnose very early stages. Ultrasound has also been a very valuable tool in diagnosing ovarian cancer and other ovarian masses.

Obstetrics and gynecology has undergone a major transformation in my lifetime. It was one specialty when I trained. Today, specialists have subspecialized in gynecologic oncology, reproductive endocrinology, perinatology, and uro-gynecology. The field of fertility has advanced tremendously in the last thirty years. Reproductive endocrinologists introduced in vitro fertilization and helped to develop new fertility drugs and surgical procedures. In vitro fertilization has also led to an increase in the multiple birth rates.

Obstetrics and gynecology continues to be a changing specialty, not only in technology, but also in the makeup of its practitioners. Surveys by the American College of Obstetricians and Gynecologists indicate that about seventy-five percent of women prefer to have a female obstetrician and gynecologist. To meet that demand, close to fifty percent of graduating obstetrical and gynecological residents are women. If the experience in Reno is indicative of what is happening nationwide, then a large percentage of female practitioners will stay in obstetrics only five to seven years after completing residency. For a multitude of reasons, they are restricting their practice to gynecology and often on a part-time basis. If this trend continues, there will not be enough obstetricians to deliver babies twenty years from now. So, who will be delivering the babies in the future? Midwives are the logical solution. The shift will be gradual, but the end result will be a few obstetricians managing groups of midwives.

One of the biggest non-technological influences in medicine has been the transformation from fee-for-service to managed care. The impact has been tremendous and has forever changed the way medicine is practiced. Third party payers and "managers" have placed themselves squarely between doctors and their patients. They have dictated what physicians can or cannot do for their patients in the guise of prior authorization mandates, shortened lengths of stay, delays in scheduling, denials of specific treatments, and refusals of claims. They have significantly reduced reimbursement to physicians for office and surgical procedures while the costs of operating a practice have continued to spiral upwards. Patient rights groups are becoming more vocal, but it is unlikely that major changes will occur.

When I came to Reno in 1968, the medical school did not exist. There were only two hospitals, Washoe and St. Mary's. Sparks Family Hospital was built in 1982, and later renamed Northern Nevada Medical Center. The first outpatient surgery center, Reno Medical Plaza, was opened about 1974, and there are now five more of these facilities. We had no CT scanners, magnetic resonance imagers, lithotripsors, medivac helicopters, or open-heart surgery facility. The changes and advances in medical care and services to the community have been tremendous. The Reno medical community has been right there on the cutting edge of using the newest technology and drugs and employing the most modern surgical techniques. The physicians are skilled and dedicated. The hospitals are top notch and the quality of care is state of the art in every way.

Reno has been an excellent place to practice medicine and raise my family. Even with the inconveniences of managed care and the rising costs of a medical education and running an office, I think medicine is and will always be a very sought after and noble profession. It is a profession one cannot help but love if he likes people. It is truly satisfying. I retired from my specialty practice in September 2000. I do surgical assisting now not only for obstetricians and gynecologists, but also for general surgeons, orthopedic surgeons, and others. I have enjoyed seeing all the different surgical techniques. I continue to learn and hope this never stops.

Notes
[1] Dr. Silas Ross was born in Nevada in 1916 and was licensed in Nevada in 1947.

[2] Dr. Clare Wolfe was born in Nebraska in 1915 and licensed in Fallon, Nevada, in 1946. Dr. Thomas Mullis was born in Texas in 1920 and licensed in Nevada in 1951. Dr. Paul Wigg was born in North Dakota in 1904 and licensed in Nevada in 1942.

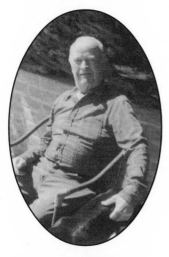
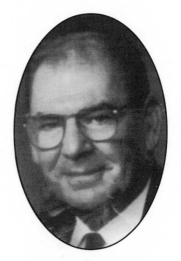

Dr. George F. Magee   Dr. Jack Talsma

8: Drs. George F. Magee and Jack Talsma, Ophthalmology

Dr. George F. Magee

Early Years and Education

I was born September 12, 1928, in Yerington, Nevada, and grew up there. My family moved to Reno when I was in my late teens. My father, George Richard, did his undergraduate and graduate work at the University of California at Berkeley and was in general practice from 1923 to 1941. He did ophthalmology training at Barnes Eye Hospital in St. Louis, Missouri.[1] My mother was a graduate of the University of Nevada in Reno. There was never any doubt that I was going to be a physician when I grew up. It was just assumed by my mother and father, two sisters, my brother, and me. My father was my creative role model in those early years, and provided me with ample encouragement along the way.

My education consisted of the following: University of Nevada (1950); Medical School at Duke University, Durham, North Carolina (1954); and internship and residency in ophthalmology at the Wilmer Institute of Ophthalmology at the Johns Hopkins Hospital (1954-1957). I considered an internal medicine practice, but ultimately chose ophthalmology because my father was an eye physician and wanted me to follow in his footsteps.

U.S. Navy

Upon graduation, I served on active duty in the navy from 1957 to 1959. I met my future wife, Jane, a social worker with the Red Cross, while I was stationed at St. Albans Hospital in Queens, New York, and we were married in 1959, the year I got out of the service. We then moved to Reno and I practiced medicine until I retired in 2001.

My three children, all daughters, were born in Reno: Susan lives in Ft. Lauderdale, Florida; Janie lives here; and Catherine lives in Washington, DC. I see them often, but not nearly as often as I would like.

Ophthalmology in Reno (Magee)

Beginning Practice

When I arrived in Reno, ophthalmological practice was comparable to starting in my military training. I took over my father's practice at the First National Bank building in downtown Reno, and the day I came to town was the day my father retired. This meant I already had all the ophthalmic equipment, instruments, and technology in place that I would need and which was available at that time. I did mostly office examinations and a small amount of surgery in that office until 1961, when I moved to West Sixth Street, where I practiced until I retired in 2001.

The eye surgery I performed was done at Washoe Medical Center and St. Mary's Hospital, and I found facilities and equipment at both hospitals quite comparable. When the freestanding surgicenter was opened at Reno Medical Plaza on Silverada Boulevard, east of downtown, I did almost all of my surgeries there from that time on. Of course, technology in the eye-care arena has improved quite a lot and all facilities in the Reno-Sparks area have kept up very well.

I don't think there have been all that many changes in medicine used in an ophthalmology practice over the years, but the technology has advanced considerably. One procedure, I recall, started out being called intracapsular cataract extraction, and that's the main surgery I did in my practice. I also did small numbers of strabismus cases and a few retinal detachment surgeries.

Ultimately, I discontinued the strabismus and retinal detachment procedures, mainly because new doctors came to town who were experts in these fields. My surgical practice was thus limited to cataract removal and later implantation of intraocular lenses. I think the discovery of this technique for implanting lenses was the most important technological event that occurred during my medical career. Patients would not have to wear those extra thick eyeglasses, and they would not have to be bedridden for up to a week after cataract removal. The bed rest requirement was changed later to twenty-four hours, and today, after the new lasik (laser-assisted keratotomy) procedure, there is no bed confinement required at all.

Cataract Surgery

Cataract removal involved making an incision and withdrawing the clouded lens intact. This usually involved making a fairly large incision and afterwards closing with large, multiple silk sutures. By the time I retired, those incisions were quite a bit smaller and fewer sutures were required. Intraocular lenses today are small and can be placed through a three-millimeter incision, which can be closed with one stitch or, in some cases, no suture at all. This has come about within the past ten years or so. Most of the ophthalmologists in town took educational courses to learn how to do these procedures, which were done as far back as 1972.

In comparison with the techniques and technology available today, those first lens implants were extremely crude, but they did work. The way that procedure is done today is far superior and probably more successful. The surgical instruments I used when I began my practice were similar to what I used before I retired, but those early instruments would be considered quite obsolete today.

Economics of Ophthalmology

Costs involved in eye surgery, I would say, are less overall today than in the early part of my practice. When I started out, doctors' fees were less, but the dollar was worth a lot more. The patient would be in the hospital for at least a week after cataract surgery. Now they go home the same day, so that cost is definitely less. Surgical fees are greater now, but so is inflation.

When I started out, my indigent patients were not charged for my services at all. I just didn't bill them. They got everything for free. Later on they had insurance available through the State Aid to the Medically Indigent program, called SAMI, and Medicare, which together covered almost all the fees so most people had little out-of-pocket expenses.

I used to enjoy going to medical and scientific meetings to keep up-to-date on what was happening in my field. Education was provided at the Nevada State Medical Association, the Washoe County Medical Society, the local hospitals, and on the regional and national ophthalmology specialty levels. My needs for learning the latest surgical advances stopped when I turned sixty-five, as I then stopped doing surgeries altogether. I shifted to an office-based practice at that time.

Lasik surgery has become very popular today, but I did not get involved in that new technology before I retired. I did do a fair amount of radial keratotomy, the precursor to lasik surgery, and I enjoyed doing those, although the results were not always predictable. In fact, lasik is a more advanced technology, more affordable, and more effective than the previous procedure.

The costs of medical liability insurance throughout my career kept creeping up, but I think these costs will probably start coming down soon, as new technologies and medical procedures reduce the incidences of malpractice suits due to better surgical results and, thus, fewer angry patients.

Well, I am sure there will be changes in technology and instrumentation as time goes by, but I can't imagine what those changes will be because I think the state of the art in ophthalmology is pretty good right now. It's interesting—I was amazed at the changes that took place in my practice over the years, and I am certain I will be amazed at the changes that will take place in the future.

Dr. Jack Talsma

Early Life and Education

Omaha, Nebraska, is where I was born (May 23, 1935) and raised, and sometime during my junior year at Lincoln High School, my friend Kim Morgan and I decided we just might want to go to medical school and become doctors. Kim and I had been school buddies since the fourth grade, and we kept medical school thoughts in our minds as we graduated from Lincoln in 1957 and the University of Nebraska in 1961. I was on the football team: "GO BIG RED!"

There was never a life-long drive to be a doctor. My father was an electrical engineer who worked for General Electric, and there weren't any medical people on either side of my family influencing me. Maybe it's the fact that I had no business experience and really wasn't interested in an engineering career that caused me to strike out on my own. I surely didn't pick the easiest of professions to enter.

Kim and I have maintained our close friendship all these years and never miss the opportunity to play in an annual invitational golf tournament back in his area, Boulder, Colorado, where he practices radiology. I've never won that tournament, and I think we must hold the record with thirty-five years of straight competition. Hope springs eternal.

Internship, Military, and Residency

After medical school at the University of Nebraska, I did my internship and had begun a surgical residency at Swedish Hospital in Seattle, Washington, when I was drafted into the air force. My career was temporarily put on hold as I watched the Cuban missile crisis unfold. Evidently Mr. Khrushchev heard I was in the military with my shotgun and he backed down.

I spent the next two years in Oklahoma City where my commanding officer, a two-year man like myself, encouraged my interest in an ophthalmology career. I always liked ophthalmology in medical school even with the little bit of exposure students were given. So, when my hitch was up, I applied and was accepted at the eye program at Baylor University and affiliated hospitals in the Texas Medical Center in Houston. I entered the program in 1964 and finished in 1967.

As I was single at that time, I worked at every job I could find. I had saved a little money and managed to put myself through internship and residency without incurring debt. Imagine that today—a doctor just out of training with no debt.

My folks helped me through medical school, but they just didn't have the resources to go beyond that. I worked summers, spring vacations, nights, holidays, and even did heavy construction work and other types of moonlighting. The weekends I had off were spent working at emergency rooms in outlying hospitals, for the grand sum of $4 an hour. So, when I worked four eight-hour shifts, I put almost $200 in my pocket. It was good money back then, and that kept me pretty well going.

After residency training, my next challenge was to look for the ideal spot to set up a practice. Doctors didn't have the Internet and scores of headhunters and brokers to locate practice opportunities during that period. New docs just had to go out and look around and find the best place to hang a shingle. I always knew I wanted to go out West; I was determined to be near mountains to hunt, fish, ski, play golf, and camp. It was the great outdoors for me; I didn't like the big city after having spent three years in Houston. It would be commonplace there to have a forty-five minutes commute wherever you wanted to go, and I didn't want to spend half my life sitting in gridlock. In addition to severe traffic congestion, Houston had high humidity and a miserable climate. There were some attractive offers to join the ophthalmology program at Baylor, but again, I just didn't want to live and work there.

So I got in my car with a list of places I might consider and I began checking them off: Albuquerque, Colorado Springs, Denver, Boulder, and then up to Cheyenne.

I liked skiing and got hooked when I was in Seattle, but I didn't want to settle there either. Aside from the big city negatives, I didn't want to live in such a rainy climate. Next it was the Portland area, then Medford, southern Oregon, and a quick look at practice opportunities in Sacramento.

I had a good friend who was in my class in medical school, Fred Boyden, who was practicing radiology in Reno, so I crossed the Sierra and visited with him for a spell.

If memory serves me correctly, it was a beautiful day in late September 1967, about seventy-five degrees, sunny, and no wind. He took me up to Lake Tahoe, we played golf, and I gave the place a good once-over, one-by-one, checking off all the things that interested me. I liked everything Reno had to offer.

There was a final swing down to Phoenix, primarily because I had a friend living in the area, but I found nothing there to change my mind.

Ophthalmology in Reno (Talsma)

The Move to Reno
Before going back to Houston and loading up a U-Haul trailer with all my possessions, I decided to call all the ophthalmologists in Reno to see what was going on. There were only five at that time: Jim Greear, Chuck Lanning, Don Mousel, Arrah Curry, and Sam Clark, and I tried as a John Doe to get an appointment for a routine eye examination. The earliest appointment possible I could get was five months away and that convinced me there was opportunity here.

Dr. Boyden encouraged me in every way to come to Reno. He thought it was a great place, and he was right. I have never for a moment regretted the decision to move here.

Association with Dr. Arrah Curry
When first in town, I met with Dr. Arrah Curry to see if he might be interested in having an associate in his office. It was an interesting interview. He asked me about my knowledge of the Seventh Day Adventist Church and I told him I thought their practitioners were God-fearing, religious people and that was about the extent of my knowledge. I always thought he just might have been doing a little evangelizing. I went to work for Arrah for $1,500 per month and thought I was rich. It was a fairly busy practice, and I would do surgeries on patients who came to me; there was never a sharing of patients. I worked there for about nine months and began to feel it was not a good fit. I was single, lived a

bachelor's life, and was perhaps less attentive to religious matters than Arrah might have thought I should be, so we parted company. Dr. Nick Landis' old office was available at 505 South Arlington Avenue and I practiced there until 1977 when my new office at 1530 East Sixth Street was built. I worked there until retirement in 2001.

Another interesting interview that comes to mind was with the Nevada Board of Medical Examiners under the leadership of Dr. Kenneth Maclean, a Reno general surgeon. That brief session was a very pleasant experience for me. I was asked some general questions about my training and background and why Reno was chosen to set up my practice. There were only a few medical questions. It's interesting how things work out. Evelyn Hilsabeck, executive director for the examining board, had a very attractive assistant named Sydney whom I met again on the slopes while skiing. Later, Sydney came to me for an eye exam and I hired her away from Evelyn and later married her.

A Solo Practice

After leaving Dr. Curry's office, things were slow and I frequently worked in the emergency room at Washoe Medical Center. Fulltime ER doctors had not yet been invented and hospital administrators usually got new guys coming to town to staff the emergency room, paying them the handsome sum of $10 an hour. So, I would work a sixteen-hour shift, like on a Saturday, and make $160 and feel good doing it. Even when I was in Arrah's office, I would work in the ER on the four o'clock to midnight shift.

My practice blossomed, and over the years I had physician associates work with me, who later developed their own practices in Reno. Gary Pomeranz worked with me for about a year, and Perry Waggoner rented space from me until he could get his own office built. I have also had three or four optometrists working in my offices over the years.

Optometrists

In the late 1970s, I was the lead ophthalmologist in town who took issue with optometrists attempting to enact laws in the Nevada legislature permitting them to do medical procedures for which they were not trained. It seemed that with each session, the optometrists gained a little more legislative authority to encroach into the practice of medicine, and there was a group of us who fought them at every turn.

I opened an office in Carson City and at Meadowwood Mall and hired optometrists to do refractions and sell eyeglasses. I also had one working in my Reno office and all this worked well until the optometry association got a law passed making it illegal for optometrists to work for anyone other than another optometrist.

The Nevada Ophthalmologic Society challenged this law, arguing that ophthalmologists were qualified to do everything optometrists could do, plus we had medical training. Well, that was our argument and it finally went to the state supreme court and we lost. It didn't take long to sell those offices to the optometrists who had been running them. The situation now is that optometrists can have financial arrangements with ophthalmologists, but they must have independent decision-making authority.

Economics of Healthcare

The economics of health and medical care is simply fascinating. For example, today cataract surgery is a $6 billion industry. The manufacture and sale of eyeglasses is an $18 billion industry. Many optometrists are pleased to take the latter and leave the former to medical doctors, and it is little wonder that many ophthalmologists have opened optical shops. Sales of sunglasses alone in our country are a $30 billion industry.

Medical Politics

I was always interested over the years in supporting organized medicine, and I attended a lot of meetings of the Washoe County Medical Society. As it happens, doctors who consistently show up at meetings wind up on committees, then on boards of directors, and eventually, if they stick around long enough, they become president. I did not run for president and was somewhat surprised to have been elected to that office. I really didn't covet all that work, but it was quite an honor and Darleen Galleron, society executive director, was so much help to me during that year.

My term as county society president coincided with a growing malpractice insurance crisis, much like what is happening in Las Vegas right now. Several doctors had talked quite openly in Nevada about going without insurance—going "bare." It seemed this worked best when the doctor had few assets—no "deep pockets." A young uninsured doctor didn't have much the courts could take from him. There is a quote that pretty much says it all: "If there are no apples on the tree, lawyers aren't going to climb it."

Somehow the thought that there were a large number of doctors in Nevada going without malpractice coverage, wound up in an article in the *Wall Street Journal,* and it was picked up by the *60 Minutes* television show.

One of the producers of *60 Minutes,* a man named Wasserman, came out and set up an interview with me. Wasserman and his crew came to my home, expecting to see a million-dollar mansion rather than my small home in Hidden Valley. They took out all of our light bulbs, replacing them with 250-watt bulbs to light up the house for the filming. They followed Sydney around, watched her fix breakfast for the kids, and watched as she burned the pancakes and bacon. But I have to say they were quite professional. The night before the interview, Sydney and I and Nevada State Medical Association CEO, Rick Pugh, and his wife, Charlotte, had dinner at Eugene's restaurant with Mr. Wasserman. We discussed how the interview would be orchestrated. CBS Correspondent Morley Safer arrived the next day and my interview was held in Hospital Administrator Carroll Ogren's office at Washoe Medical Center.

The research done by Mr. Wasserman on this issue, both with doctors and lawyers in Reno, was fair and balanced. I thought my answer, when asked by Mr. Safer, "Dr. Talsma, don't you think lawyers have principles?" was appropriate then and now. I replied, "Yes, they certainly do have principles and here they are." Then I waved several dollar bills in the air. I have always thought that comment was the highlight of that particular *60 Minutes* segment.

I thought seriously about going through the "chairs" on the state medical association level, but decided against it because of the time commitment that would be required. My feeling at the time was that no matter what presidents of voluntary organizations do, half the people are glad and half the people are mad. That was not needed at that stage of my career. In retrospect, I feel I was wrong in thinking that way, and I wish I had gone forward with the state association presidency. I think the positives would have greatly outweighed the negatives and it would have been a great experience.

State-of-the-Art in Reno

I remember when I came to Reno, basically everything I was taught and all the surgical techniques I learned in my training were in place here. It is remarkable that so very little of that knowledge and technology is in play here today. State-of-the-art technology today has proved so much better than what we had back in the late 1960s. There have been quantum leaps forward in ophthalmology, like in radiology where there have also been tremendous advances. Cardiology is another specialty that has experienced fantastic advances. When I opened my practice, I performed cataract surgery, which is probably the most common surgery ophthalmologists do. I opened up half the eye (180 degrees) took out the cataract, and used ten sutures to close the incision. Patients were in the hospital for about a week with their heads immobilized between sand-bags the entire time, and I saw them everyday.

Cataract Surgery

Gradually we cut down the hospital stays to about three days and gave patients these really thick glasses, which offered no peripheral vision. Successful surgery assured only straight-ahead vision with a twenty-five percent image magnification. Depth perception was really thrown off. Another option was the use of hard contact lenses, which gave relatively normal vision. Senior citizens usually don't have an easy time with contacts. Many older people develop a little tremor, plus there was very limited vision when the contact lenses were removed. Therefore, contact lenses were not a good answer for patients over seventy, but it was an option and, in most cases, it did give better vision.

In 1975, we began placing the first intraocular lenses. This was a great advance for ophthalmologists. Those first lenses, back in the late 1960s, were not perfect and it took quite a while before they were finally approved by the FDA for use. They slid around and there were no good means of stabilizing them to maintain vision. The English worked out most of the bugs, and after about ten years, Americans started working on them, and they began to get better. Every month there were new and different types of lenses coming out, in attempts to solve the problem of instability, which was eventually solved.

Then a procedure called phacoemulsification came along. The lens itself is composed of three main parts. It has a capsule, cortex, and a nucleus. In cataract surgery we were removing the capsule and cortex, and in the process removed the entire lens. With phacoemulsification, a little hole is cut in the capsule to take out the cataract while leaving the capsule. Then the lens is slid into the already-anchored capsule—a few small sutures and that was it.

There weren't too many advances in the 1980s and only a few in the early 1990s. There were lens improvements, smaller incisions, and incision-sealing substances that required no suturing at all. Earlier procedures that might have taken about forty minutes could now be done in twelve minutes using only topical eye drops rather than general anesthesia. There was a female golfer recently who had this procedure done and began a three-day tournament the next day. She won the tournament too! So, essentially, phacoemulsification has been a big advancement.

It is possible that physicians in all specialties are becoming victims of their own successes—take Medicare, for example. They used to authorize $2,400 for cataract surgery and pay eighty percent of that. Patients would have to pay for lost time in the hospital, deductibles, copays, and those thick glasses. Now we have gotten so damn good with this procedure, doing it so quickly without requiring expensive hospitalizations and medical rounds, that we have saved the Medicare program millions and millions of dollars over the years. By way of thanks for this advanced technology and medical skill, cataract surgery reimbursement has been reduced to $750, and they fuss at us for not spending as much time with our patients. There is a move now to reduce reimbursement to $500. This may force ophthalmologists to specialize only in cataract surgery, doing hundreds of them a day to make a living.

If we are just going to be doing one or two cataracts a week, we are better off staying in the office and doing refractions. We would make more money selling glasses, you know, being an optometrist, than we would as an ophthalmologist.

This is a case where technology has backfired on us. It just seems that Medicare and other third-party payers rewarded us for using ancient technology, and, as soon as technology improved, we were economically punished. It's something like the reward for perfection is punishment, and it makes me shake my head a lot.

Laser Surgery

Lasers came along next and eye physicians use them for all sorts of things. They are used in the retina for diabetic retinopathy, retinal tears, retinal detachments, and repairing retinal hemorrhages. The argon laser, or krypton laser, has specific value in treating many of those problems and is also used in treating glaucoma. There are "hot" and "cold" lasers in use today, and surgery has come into its own in the last five years. Lasik surgery has created a tremendous amount of excitement and is considered a major step forward.

Laser technology was not advanced inexpensively, and its use today is not inexpensive. It costs about half a million dollars to have the equipment in the office, and, consequently, it's not in every doctor's office. Fees for corrective lasik surgery are high, and, although fees have come down somewhat, they may not come down much more. One-time cost for using this equipment are about $200 in gases, royalties, and so forth, and those costs are likely to increase over time; but success rates for lasik surgery are approaching ninety-nine percent with only minor complications. That is remarkable.

Radial Keratotomy

Lasik surgery and that technology all but eliminated a procedure called radial keratotomy (RK) that showed up in the 1980s. I was the first doctor in Reno to do this procedure. It created a lot of patient complaints and overall success rates using RK were not nearly as high as when physicians began using lasik technology today. My last RK procedure was done in 1995.

When radial keratotomy first came in, I thought the future of ophthalmology was going to be in refractive surgery, and since then, I've done about two thousand of them. At the time I thought RK worked, but I thought there has to be something better. There are too many cases in which there is only a seventy-eighty percent result, and there are complications. I thought significant advances in refractive surgeries were going to be pretty slow. I think I was right on target with that.

When eye doctors reattach retinas that have been dislodged, such as those that occur with boxing injuries, they use "hot" or "heat" lasers that literally "spot welds" the retina back into place. We actually fry those tissues together, and there is some tissue destruction, but it is usually on the periphery, and, therefore, vision is not affected much.

Eye Glasses Technology

There hasn't been much breakthrough in glasses. They talk about these blue blocker sunglasses, and studies have been done by our military using aviator glasses. After spending $1,000,000 in research, they concluded that sunglasses don't do any harm. Actually, they don't do any good either. It has been proven that the more one wears sunglasses, the more eyes get used to subdued light, and sunglasses become addictive. Now there are times when they are definitely indicated, like while skiing and playing water sports in places where there is glare. Some glasses keep out more rays than others, but the damage caused by sunrays is really overblown. If UV rays caused severe damage, every rancher, farmer, roofer, construction worker, logger, and golfer would have cataracts. Practically none of the golfers wear sunglasses and those who wear only billed caps are exposed to UV rays. There is no higher incidence of cataracts among people who don't wear sunglasses than the rest of the population. Most eyeglasses don't filter out UV rays, but sunglass manufactures neglect to mention this in order to have a marketing tool.

Advances in Ophthalmology

I don't see any fantastic advances coming down the pike in cataract surgery anytime in the very near future. There will be advances, but they will be quite slow. In fact, there have been refinements and fine-tuning, but the basic technology hasn't changed much in the past thirty years.

The biggest problem that ophthalmologists see in their offices today is macular degeneration. It affects about fifteen percent of people over sixty-five, and its very, very slow onset is deceptive. Since it has genetic causative roots, it may well be sometime before successful treatments can be realized. Retinal tissue re-growth may be a solution, but retinal tissue is central nervous system tissue and once it is dead, it is gone. This will be the next big challenge for eye doctors.

On the economic front, it is interesting that Canadian ophthalmologists were approved for LASIK surgery three years before we were, and, consequently, thousands of American went to Canada for that surgery. It would be quite hard to estimate how much revenue was shipped to our Canadian medical colleagues, but physicians there did excellent work. I referred many patients there and would not be afraid to go there myself if I need lasik surgery. It is interesting, too, that lasik work is still considered "cosmetic" by all insurance companies. This has its advantages as far as economics is concerned. Patients are ready, willing, and able to pay up front for this procedure, and physicians do not have to deal with insurers and all those "managed care" people.

I am thankful to have time today to reflect on my medical career, the changes that have taken place in technology, in reimbursement mechanisms, in expectations of patients, in the roles of hospitals, and to muse on what the future holds for my profession.

I know that I have enjoyed my work and my life and I have certainly enjoyed my time away from my work. Africa has been one of my chief diversions over the years, and Sydney and I have enjoyed many trips there. Sometimes we hunted, sometimes we fished, and sometimes we just enjoyed the magnitude of it all. It is said you can never go to Africa just once. We even thought about opening an eye clinic there, but after thinking it over—doing forty cataracts every day, seven days a week, the idea sort of slipped away. Maybe if I were twenty years younger I would consider it.

Will I keep my hand in ophthalmology? I honestly don't think so. I have enjoyed so much of medicine, the physician friends I have made, the patient friends I have made, the medical challenges I have faced, and the joy of preventing blindness and creating sight where there was none before. All that is in my mind and in my heart and to try to make that continue forever would not be possible.

There have been parts of the practice of medicine that have not been all that enjoyable. The medical malpractice problem began in the early part of my practice and is prominent today. When managed care came in, I knew that the practice of medicine would be changed and would become less enjoyable. Yet, it too, was endured. Physicians have had to endure under some quite stringent conditions, and I suppose that will never improve. Changes have been everywhere—medical colleagues have become medical competitors and the practice of medicine has become a business of the first order. Still, it was fun, challenging, and rewarding in so many ways

Notes

[1] Dr. George R. Magee was born in California in 1896 and licensed in Yerington in 1923.

9: Dr. Charles McCuskey, Orthopedic Surgery

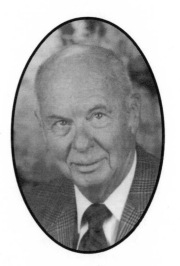

Dr. Charles McCuskey

Early Life and Nevada Connections

I was born May 17, 1932, in Rochester, Minnesota, but I grew up in southern California. However, my folks had a ranch up in Elko, Nevada, where I spent a lot of summers. During World War II, we lived in San Francisco where my dad, an anesthesiologist, was stationed at Letterman Hospital.

My earliest connection with Nevada was with Dr. Fred Anderson of Reno, who was a surgeon at Letterman Hospital and a good friend of my folks. I got to know Fred pretty well. My dad had met several doctors in northern Nevada as a result of having been invited to speak at the Reno Surgical Society.

My dad was a friend of a prominent Los Angeles surgeon named Arnold Stevens who was the personal physician for singer Bing Crosby. At the time, Crosby had a big spread in Elko County, which was a very popular place for southern Californians, although I never knew the reason. The Crosby spread had thousands of acres and that made property surrounding it far too expensive. The ranch dad eventually bought was purchased from the Marble family, the W. T. Jenkins Company, and was thirty-seven hundred acres. I met a lot of the people who worked for Bing Crosby, but I never met him.

The other Nevada connection was my cousin, a dentist in Fallon. After he finished dental school in 1946, he moved to Fallon and I would spend a month or so in the summer with him. Dad bought a ranch there after selling the Elko County place.

The McCuskey family men, traditionally, were ministers, physicians, and dentists. There was a whole tribe of doctors back in West Virginia with the name of McCuskey, and another tribe of Methodist ministers, which meant none of them drank or smoked. The ones that drank and smoked, I guess, became doctors. That's how that worked.

There are three Charles F. McCuskey, M.D.s in our family and my father was one of the early anesthesia specialists in the country and a founder of the American Board of Anesthesiology. He practiced in Los Angeles most of his career and moved to the Fallon ranch when he retired. One of his accomplishments was being responsible for Reno's first anesthesiologist, Dr. Bill O'Brien, moving to Reno.

My Dad, Pioneer Anesthesiologist

Dad was one of the first M.D. anesthesiologists in the Los Angeles area. During World War II, he moved to Letterman Hospital in San Francisco, where he was chief of the anesthesia department and began a short training program for newly commissioned physicians. They received anesthesia training at Letterman in order to go to the Pacific area for the invasion of Japan. They were stationed on various Pacific islands to take care of the wounded. When these doctors returned after the war, some of them went to Los Angeles County Hospital for more anesthesia training. Dad was head of the staff there, and one of the men he trained was Dr. Bill O'Brien. When it came time for him to go into practice, Bill asked dad, "Where do you think I ought to go?" Dad encouraged him to go to Reno, as both had known Dr. Fred Anderson when they were working at Letterman.

When Bill arrived in Reno, there were some general practitioners doing anesthesia, but that changed as more anesthesiologists moved to Reno. As more anesthesiologists came to Reno, they were quickly overwhelmed and asked my dad to help out three days a week. He and mom were living in Fallon by then and agreed to come to Reno. They initially stayed at the Holiday or the Riverside Hotels, but when more coverage was needed, the doctors rented an apartment for mom and dad on Hill Street, where they would come and spend the whole week. He was practicing in town when I moved here.

Education

After high school I graduated from Stanford University. While there, I decided to pursue a medical career and was accepted and completed my medical degree at the University of Southern California School of Medicine. However, I really wanted to be a cowboy, but my hay fever and asthma made that line of work impractical.

In medical school I took an interest in becoming an oncologist, and that was before anybody knew what an oncologist was. In my senior year I came down with a serious illness called post-influenza meningomyelitis, which caused me to miss six weeks of my surgical clerkship and set me back quite a bit. I began to think of oncology and surgery, as it was one of the key management tools for tumors. I decided to take a surgical internship at the Bellevue Hospital in New York City. I thought training there would be helpful and give me a chance to see the East Coast and the rest of the world.

During my training Dr. Jane Wright, who we never hear of historically, was doing chemotherapy on cancer patients on our service. As interns we were responsible for hanging the IV and administering the medicine. This turned out to be so depressing because all of the people were dying. They would die about the time we hung up those IVs. Chemotherapy is standard treatment for a lot of cancers now, but in the 1950s and '60s they were experimenting with it to see what it could do. Dr. Wright was basically working with terminal patients who had agreed to try these drugs. She was getting some results and some of the tumors would regress. Many of the patients were so sick that they didn't survive the fevers and reactions from the medications.

Decision to Pursue Orthopedics

While in New York, however, I had fun doing surgery, and I spent time on a fracture service, which really appealed to me. Orthopedics was pretty much an open specialty at that time; most fractures were done by general surgeons in New York. On the other hand, I knew out West fractures were done by orthopedists. There and then I decided orthopedics and not oncology was for me. I met my future wife, Angie, who was a nurse in the Bellevue Hospital pediatric emergency room, and we were married in New York during my training. After two years in New York, I decided to return to Los Angeles for my orthopedic residency at the county hospital.

Orthopedic Surgery in Reno

The Move to Reno

I had ties to Nevada and wanted to show Angie the area. We had a little Borgwald automobile at the time and an even smaller apartment. We loaded the contents of the apartment, except for the couch, into that little German car and headed west. That poor old car over-heated going up the hills those hot summer days. I had to turn on the heater to cool it down some, but I was determined to show her Nevada. We plotted a course through Salt Lake, Elko, Reno, and on to Los Angeles, but we started to run short of time so our course was modified and we headed southwest, spending a night in Ely. We stayed at the Old Nevada Hotel, and Angie watched this old man in Levi's throwing $100 bills on the craps table and said, "That poor man, he's throwing away his whole living." I pointed out to her that the poor little old man might have millions. Then we came down through Tonopah and that was a desolate road. Even today it's a desolate road with its wide-open vistas. Angie said, "This is terrible. There is nothing here. This is awful." She complained all the way across the state. Years later Angie, my three kids, my dad, and I went on a camping trip to the old ranch in Elko, which had been sold by then, and we came home by way of Tonopah on that same stretch of road. Angie said, "Boy those rocks are so pretty. Isn't that mountain gorgeous!" Nevada had really grown on her.

At the end of my orthopedic surgery training at LA County Hospital, we moved to Reno. I had taken a look at Phoenix and Tucson but after only a short visit to those places I came to realize all the orthopedists there hated each other. There were two or three groups in each area and on visiting one group they told you how bad the other guys were and the next group told you how bad the first guys were. I didn't care for that atmosphere at all. I had visited Reno and talked with Drs. Jimmy Herz, Jack Sargent, Bill Teipner, and Hal Halvorson and was very impressed with how encouraging they were. The doctors later named their group the "Reno Orthopedic Clinic, (ROC)," but they didn't have that title when I came to town. They also agreed to generously share emergency room call, which was very important for a new guy just starting out. I sort of filled a niche being a young solo practitioner. The reception I got at this very first meeting with my Reno colleagues convinced me to come to Reno.

Starting Practice

Once in Reno, obtaining staff privileges at the two hospitals was not as stringent as it would become in later years. If you got privileges to do surgery, you could do any kind of surgery you wanted regardless of your training. Eventually, when the hospitals came out with privilege cards, I saw that I had privileges to do thyroidectomies and all sorts of other procedures I was not qualified to do.

I opened my office in Dr. Frank Rueckl's building at 890 Mill Street and four of the first five patients I saw in that office were referrals from the Herz, Sargent, Teipner, and Halvorson group. By the end of six weeks I was as busy as I could be.

Many doctors didn't choose orthopedics back then because it generally involved taking care of patients over a very long period of time and they didn't like that. I personally liked it. I'd go along with my treatment plan for months or a year before I might see progress on some of my patients, like post-polio cases and the rheumatoid arthritics. Some of them were never actually cured, but they were my patients until they either got tired of me or died.

Trauma was probably the most common thing orthopedists saw in their practices, and somebody pointed out that orthopedists follow their patients through their aging process. The Greek translation for the term "orthopedics" is "straight children." We see a lot of children with congenital-dislocated hips, clubfeet, and cerebral palsies, and all these are long-term problems. When I applied for the residency at the LA County Hospital, orthopedics was not a popular specialty. Two years before I applied, five doctors applied for six positions. A year before I applied, six doctors applied for a position there and got one. The year I applied, thirty-six out of seventy-two applicants were interviewed; all of a sudden orthopedics became popular and I don't quite know what triggered that. Every year thereafter they were taking just the top one percent of the medical school classes, so I kind of sneaked in the back door.

State-of-the-Art in Reno

Reno was state-of-the-art in imaging technology, but imaging technology at that time was just starting. All we really had were x-rays. We did pantopaque myelograms, and as it turned out, those caused serious complications. Dye would be injected into the spinal canal to outline lumbar discs, and the dye would sometimes cause a reaction. There was an argument at the time whether orthopedists shouldn't just operate using the clinical picture alone. CT scanners or MRI imagers would come along much later.

Almost everything we did changed during the years I was in practice. The way we treated fractures took a major turn at least twice. For a while, we didn't do open reductions. If a femur was broken, the patient's leg hung in traction for six or eight weeks and was then put in a spica cast. The types of nails and devices we used during operation on broken hips all changed over time, and as the imaging got faster and better, it became a lot easier to nail a hip because we could get a bunch of x-rays in a hurry. Earlier we had to wait seven or eight minutes for a tech to develop the film and drag it into the operating room. Sometimes changes and new pictures were necessary, and the x-ray lag time repeated itself. It was a very tedious process.

There was naturally some overlapping and a little competition about which specialty was best at lumbar disc procedures, but I was well trained to do them and there were always enough cases to go around. Drs. Ernie Mack, Adolf Rosenauer, and Chuck Fleming, were the neurosurgeons in town when I arrived, and we all helped each other a lot.

When I arrived in Reno in 1964, the nearest orthopedist to the east was in Salt Lake City; to the north there were one or two in Medford, Oregon; to the west there was one man in Auburn and several in Sacramento; but the closest orthopedist to the south was in Lancaster in southern California. I got patients from Elko and Ely but others went to Salt Lake. Patients from Ely came to Reno because Drs. Walter Quinn and Noah Smernoff had practiced there before they moved to Reno and their patients followed them. Winnemucca patients came here because they followed Dr. Frank Rueckl. I had patients from Lakeview (Oregon), Lake Tahoe, Susanville, and all over, so our population base was pretty large.

Orthopedists in Reno rarely referred cases to other areas, but there was one disease we generally did refer out and that was malignant bone tumors. To be honest, there were only two of those in my whole career that I sent out, as they were quite rare. We were as good as any place in the country, and even in the event of surgical complications, we had backup right here to handle them.

As the new imaging equipment came to town, I became trained to read my own films and MRIs and had excellent backup from the radiologists in town. We would both read them. Because orthopedists know the underlying anatomy probably better than radiologists, I think we would sometimes see things they didn't see.

I think St. Mary's is state-of-the-art today, but when I came to town, Saints really wasn't up to speed when I had a really ill person. The food there was always good, and doctors and patients were treated better, so a lot of patients preferred to be treated at St. Mary's. St. Mary's was not a twenty-four hour hospital back then, and if an EKG was needed in the middle of the night, a tech would be called in to do one. If somebody needed an x-ray in the middle of the night, a tech would be called in to take a picture. When I first arrived, St. Mary's was not state-of-the-art by any stretch of the imagination.

During the early days of my career in Reno, the St. Mary's administrator was Sister Seraphine, and she did a good job running the facility. When the emergency room was first opened, not everybody was in favor because it meant there would be two emergency rooms and we were on-call twice as often. It was convenient to only have one ER to cover, and if you had a really sick patient, you wanted that patient to be at Washoe.

Drs. Claire Harper and Jack Becker were also practicing in town, and I think they were the first two "bone men" in Reno; there were other orthopedists who came to town as time went on. I remember Dr. Jerry Dales came on the scene and associated with Jack Becker, but that didn't work out too well and he went solo. Later, Dr. Glenn Miller arrived and opened his solo practice. It's interesting how medical groups are formed to help out with the "on-call" situation. I know some independent doctors who complained about the phone ringing, knowing they would have to go to work; then they complained because the phone didn't ring and they wondered what was wrong with the phone.

Osteoarthritis

When I started practice, there were about three procedures available to alleviate osteoarthritis of the hip. One procedure was osteotomy, in which the bone is cut and weight bearing is shifted off the arthritic hip by taking the lever arm off the hip abductors. This gave the patient a pretty bad limp and a short leg, but it seemed to help the pain. Another procedure was cup arthroplasty, in which both sides of the joint would be ground down and a metal cup would be inserted. The third thing we could do was insert a metal ball. None of these procedures were very successful.

Another procedure we performed was total hip joint replacement, which required out-of-area training but was a major advancement for orthopedists. We had to take a course to get permission from the Federal Food and Drug Administration to administer polymethylmethacrylate (PMMA).[1] The course was given at UC Davis, where I assisted Dr. Paul Lipscomb on a case or two. This surgery was not much more complex than a cup arthroplasty, but it was different. Today this procedure is quite good, but it does have its complications. When we initially started doing them, the mortality rate was three to five percent. Pulmonary emboli created major problems. Some people would have a reaction to the PMMA, which I still don't quite understand. The anesthesiologists began to anticipate problems and really hydrated the patients beforehand; we didn't seem to have any problems, but at the start there were complications.

Knee Injuries

A huge change during the years I practiced was the introduction of the arthroscope. Previous to this there was no way to look inside a joint. We made a hole—a big hole—looked in and then had to sew it up. Arthroscopes were a huge advance, particularly in knee surgery. Now they are also using them in shoulder surgery. Orthopedists had to learn how to use these instruments through training and on-the-job experience.

Skiing has always been a very popular sport in our area and back then boots and bindings were not the state-of-the-art they are today. I remember poor bindings kept me busy all winter, as I saw a lot of broken ankles. There were no orthopedists up at the ski areas, so all of the patients came down to Reno. Being on call on winter weekends was quite a busy time for orthopedists in town. I remember seeing fifty patients the first day of the Junior Ski Program. They were bringing them by the ambulance load from Sky Tavern. Other doctors working in the emergency room would scream because of the caseload, but many injuries were not breaks, they were sprains and the patients would be sent on their way. Ligament surgery was not a big thing until about the time I finished my residency. If you tore your ligaments back then, the state-of-the-art treatment was, "Here's your knee brace." Nobody had the techniques then to repair ligaments, and even after we had the techniques, results weren't all that good. Treatment and therapy in this area have made real strides.

The major advance in ligament repair has been the reconstruction of anterior cruciate ligaments (ACL). A lot of people have ruptured an ACL skiing, and as a result of this, bindings and boots were improved. We then began seeing less sprained ankles and more fractured tibias. It seems today orthopedists are seeing more knee injuries. Some of them are the results of skiers stressing their knees a lot more than they should.

Shoulder Surgery

Torn rotator cuffs in the shoulder were numerous in my practice, from the very beginning. They were always common and easily diagnosed, but the techniques for repairing them were not too good. The problem was acute in senior citizens, and orthopedists would just be honest with these older patients by telling them, "If you are sixty, forget it." That's the group of people who tear their rotator cuffs most often. They were painful but not fatal, and patients had to live with them.

Over the years, better imaging helped us in making better diagnoses. With the arthroscope, we could go in and see the size of the tear and make a much smaller incision than previously. Techniques for repairing the cuff have also steadily improved.

Drug Therapy

The first non-steroidal anti-inflammatory drug, or NSAID, was aspirin, which was introduced by the early Greeks. Aspirin came from willow bark and has been steadily improved over the years. NSAIDs actually have curative value in conditions like bursitis, but not for osteoarthritis. We had Butazolidin and Tandearil when I was in residency and both were pretty good, but they had some terrible side effects, like aplastic anemia.

That didn't happen often, but if you were the patient who got it and died, that was not a good result.

Probably the biggest improvement in my practice occurred when the infectious disease doctors came up with drugs to combat orthopedic infections. Earlier, here infections were almost impossible to cure, but they did an excellent job handling complex antibiotics. They understood the drug sensitivities involved, and I was very happy for their help with infections in my patients.

Most of the NSAIDs have adverse side effects. I've taken one of the newer drugs myself, a cyclooxygenase 2 inhibitor (Cox 2 inhibitor), but I don't think it has the effectiveness of some of the others.

An area of ongoing research is cartilage repair: implantation of cartilage, cartilage growth stimulators, and drugs along those lines have recently been introduced. How good they are? I can't say.

Physical Therapy, Osteopaths, and Chiropractors

Physical therapy was an established profession long before I started my career, as was the medical profession of physical therapy specialists, who are called physiatrists. Both of these groups worked under supervision, usually of an orthopedic surgeon, and I think that was a good system. I always encouraged my patients that needed physical therapy to do most of the work themselves. The physical therapists could encourage them and motivate them, but my patients had to do the actual therapy. As I understand it, physical therapists today are working to gain total independence from physicians.

Chiropractors have been independent from physicians the beginning. The Palmer College of Chiropractice located in Glendale, California, was only a six-month course. On the other hand, osteopathy dates back to the old theory that troubles in the spine cause illnesses, like asthma, for example. Osteopaths are a different situation as they have modernized their schools and are now also designated as M.D.s because their training is equivalent. It had been recognized earlier that the old osteopathic theories were not holding up. Those early principles were based on flawed logic, but it was as good as any logic that had existed before the twentieth century.

Rehabilitation after having total knee surgery can be very painful and exhausting; the CPM machine is very effective in the recovery process, but it, too, can be uncomfortable. I had a patient who needed both knees replaced, but after the first surgery decided not to have the second one done even though he really needed it. I felt very badly this old gentleman elected not to go forward. He had this beautiful, perfectly straight leg and this terribly bowed crooked one, and I never quite understood why he didn't get the second one done. He simply thought it hurt too much.

Organized Medicine

I first got involved in organized medicine when I was elected chief of surgery at St. Mary's Hospital. The funny thing is I didn't know I was supposed to go to executive committee meetings. Chief of staff Dr. John Ervin finally came to me and said, "You've got to come to the executive committee meeting tonight, we're kicking a doctor off staff." And so, I went to the executive committee and listened to the story and voted to kick the man off the staff. We asked him if he had anything to say and he pleaded, "Gee, I wish you wouldn't do that," and that was the end of it. Now, when you go to kick somebody off staff, you have forty lawyers intervening.

One of the very enjoyable groups I belonged to was the Reno Surgical Society, and in the early years "Reno Surg" was a very good academic organization with monthly meetings, medical speakers, and a yearly scientific assembly. It evolved into a monthly supper club meeting and I dropped out.

I used to go to the county medical society meetings on a regular basis. It was almost a requirement and they were fun too. I remember a fight one night, but that was an exception. There was always something medical and political to talk about. I became active, but not all that active, on society committees and things like that, and I stayed pretty much up on the business at the hospitals. Over the years I served on several hospital groups, such as vice chief of staff, chairman of the orthopedics department, and chief of medical records, which I disbanded at Washoe for over seven years until the accreditation commission found out about it. This disbanding did save a lot of meetings. Eventually, I served two years as chief of staff at Washoe.

As president of the Washoe County Medical Society, I headed up the delegation to the state association house of delegates, and I took an interest in medical politics, which eventually led to my serving as president in 1994. As state association president, I fought the battle doctors are fighting right now on tort reform and got talked into running for the state assembly against the co-chairman of the judiciary committee, David Humke, a lawyer who gave doctors a hard time during the 1993 legislative process. That was an interesting experience and, in hindsight, I am not sorry I lost. While I do not plan to ever run for public office again, walking the neighborhood streets was a fascinating experience and I had some interesting sociological revelations.

The election was not close. I spent about fifteen thousand dollars while my opponent spent over sixty thousand dollars. His TV spots had testimonials from people like former Congresswoman Barbara Vucanovich and Washoe District Attorney Dick Gammick telling how wonderful he was and how much he was needed in the assembly. The day after the election, I called David Humke to congratulate him on running such a clean campaign and he was speechless. I think he kept waiting for me to drop the next shoe or something at the end of the campaign and that didn't happen. The day after the call I got a note from Dave saying, "I am sorry, I was totally inappropriate, I was just speechless. After all my elections never has my opponent called me to congratulate me and I appreciate it. If there is anything I can do for you, please let me know."

The Future in Orthopedics

Looking ahead I am not sure I can even imagine what is coming down the "pike." In 1900 a doctor could not have envisioned or imagined all the changes that would take place in the twentieth century. He would not have had a clue. I do think, in addition to developing new cartilage growth material and creating advances with stem cell research, which will be impressive, researchers are going to introduce better materials for the total joint replacement and better prostheses will come along. There are big companies now working to improve hip prostheses that look promising. A while back there were researchers working with metal-on-metal prostheses and it was a disaster. But, as time went by, they revisited that technology and worked out some of the bugs. Now they are finding that metal-on-metal has better wear characteristics.

I suspect there will be continuous changes in antibiotics, but who knows whether they will be better or not. It may well be that germs are going to adapt to those, too. Certainly major improvements have occurred in the treatment of bone cancers, for example, osteogenic sarcoma. I remember comments when I was a resident that if a patient was alive five years after the original diagnosis of bone cancer, somebody had made the wrong diagnosis. Today, doctors are showing a good fifty percent survival rate at five years with no evidence of disease, so major progress has been made. Who knows where we are going next. We can hope, too, that researchers some place will find the missing enzyme in the genetic field that will eventually lead to curing rheumatoid arthritis.

Only one of my children, Charles F. McCuskey III, elected to go into medicine. He is married to a transplant nephrologist in Texas with no expectations of ever moving to Reno. I have four other children: one is a lawyer, one is a schoolteacher, one is studying to be a veterinary technician, and another raises children and goats.

Raising my family in Reno has been an adventure. Angie and I have enjoyed our lives here, made tons of friends, and have gotten as active in civic and community work as we have wanted. Among the things we did was help found and serve the local volunteer fire department in Hidden Valley. The medical community has been just great, my career couldn't have been any better, and I am enjoying my retirement ever so much.

Notes
[1] This is sometimes referred to as glue and is a chemical that hardens and holds the prosthesis in place.

10: Dr. Bud West, Otolaryngology

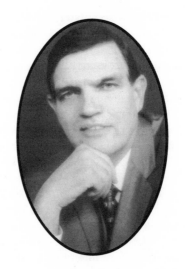

Dr. Bud West

Raised on a Farm

I was born in a little town called Spanish Fork, Utah, on May 22, 1943. The town is located in central Utah, near Provo, where my family had a small but productive farm and cattle ranch near Utah Lake. We raised a lot of row crops like peas, lima beans, corn, and sugar beets, and in our pasture we raised hay and grain for the cattle. My mom and dad also raised children. There were seven of us, and I was right in the middle with two younger brothers and a younger sister; two older brothers and an older sister. Things were lean in those days, and we grew up in meager circumstances, but we never considered ourselves to be poor even though we had very little.

My dad did a good job of providing for all the kids. Even though he didn't have much education beyond high school, he felt the importance of education and made sure we had projects on the farm, which mostly involved raising and selling cattle and sheep that could make some money. We put money aside for college, and when we started college, we were all set.

Education

All through high school my dream was to go into veterinary medicine. A good friend and I went all the way through high school and undergraduate school together. We both wanted to be vets, and while at Utah State University, we both applied to veterinary school after just three years of study. Back then that necessitated taken extremely heavy class loads each semester. On a dare, we decided we would also put in applications for medical school. The University of Utah School of Medicine acceptance letters came about two weeks before we were to hear from the veterinary schools, so we accepted the offer. Later we both got accepted to vet school, but we decided being medical doctors would be a better deal. That's how it happened. I would become the first medical doctor in the family, as far as I know, but one of my brothers did become an orthodontist and another has his doctorate in sociology.

I started medical school in 1964 and graduated in 1968. I got married the second year. Actually my wife to be, Joyce, and I started courting at Utah State, and when I went to the University of Utah School of Medicine, we began a long distance relationship. My first year of med school was a real challenge for me in several ways. Because I was accepted into medical school after only three years of undergraduate work, there was no time to take the required calculus courses. I had to take those my first year of med school in addition to the regular med school curriculum. Starting medical school, catching up on math, and dating Joyce long-distance made for a very challenging first year. In addition, and to compound things, I developed infectious mononucleosis my first semester and became quite ill. Before it was even diagnosed, I was out of school for two weeks. The dean called me into his office after mid-term exams and said, "Do you want to start over next year?" I convinced him I was OK and could catch up, and I did.

Residency and Public Health Service

It seemed like from my first day in medical school I had already made up my mind to become an ear, nose, and throat (ENT) doctor and I never had any thoughts of being anything else.

For my otolaryngology residency training I went to the University of Oregon in Portland, and I worked at the four separate hospitals up there on the hill. At the time I was accepted into my residency program, I had been given a military deferment since the Vietnam conflict was going on. After completing my residency training, I would pay back for my deferment with two years of service in the public health. I served those two years at U.S. Public Health Service hospital in the Indian Health Service in Phoenix, Arizona. I got acquainted with Reno because I was flying here about every three months, then driving down to the ENT clinic at the Schurz Indian Colony near Walker Lake. I consulted with some of the ENT doctors in the Reno community through correspondence and by phone regarding my Native American patients, and they provided necessary follow-up when I had to go back to the Phoenix area.

Otolaryngology in Reno

Move to Reno

When my two-year hitch was up in Arizona, I moved to Reno and found it to be a very progressive medical community. Some of the ENT doctors here in 1975 were Tom Kavanaugh, Dick Cavell, John Brophy, Scottie Marshall, Ralph Coppola, Olin Moulton, who was double trained in ENT and eye, and Joe Elia who picked up his ENT training in the military.[1]

Many of the basic procedures we do today were done back then, like correcting deviated septa and draining fluid buildup from behind children's eardrums. These were the bread and butter of the specialty at the time. When we put tubes in the eardrums and did tonsillectomies and adenoidectomies (T&A), the techniques we used were basically the same ones we use today. There have been vast improvements in instruments, however, and imaging technology has changed quite a bit. For example, today I do tonsils using lasers and adenoids using a microdebrider, which is an instrument that sucks and cuts. I use CT scans to help make important diagnoses. This technology gives a lot more precision and patients recover quicker. ENT doctors still use a lot of the standard techniques and surgical procedures used years ago.

Age of Antibiotics

The whole antibiotic phenomenon was just mushrooming when I was in med school and residency. The cephalosporins were introduced during that time and drugs like Clindamycin and aminoglycocides were being introduced and used in Reno. Prior to about 1960, penicillin and the sulfonamides were the main drugs of choice for treating infections, and we have come a long way since then.

There has been a revolution in antibiotic therapy. Drugs we use today like the quinolones were unheard of at that time, and even most of the macrolytes, except for just plain erythromycin, were not around. Along with these miracle drugs have come drug-resistant strains of organisms such as *Streptococcal pneumonia* and *Hemophilus influenza bacillus*. Drug companies have done a pretty good job of keeping one step ahead of these organisms, but there is evidence today that the battle is being lost.

Drug Marketing to Patients

A fairly recent phenomenon that has occurred in the last few years is that of drug companies marketing directly to patients. I see more and more of it in my practice. Patients are coming to me requesting prescriptions for this or that which they have seen on TV. I think that's where patients see most of the advertisements, and we see many patients who ask for drugs they have seen advertised on TV, the Internet, or heard about from their friends. According to the drug reps, we may well be seeing more of that in the future. After all, drug companies know best how their products should be marketed.

The formularies that insurance and managed care companies have developed have also handcuffed physicians quite a lot. The drug of choice, the absolutely best drug for my patients may not be in those formularies, and if it isn't, the patient will have to pay a hefty price to get it. In my field, particularly in treating allergies, most of my patients will take what I prescribe for them, and I warn them that there is a lot of misinformation regarding not only drugs, but surgical techniques, as well.

When I came to town in 1975, St. Mary's and Washoe Medical Center were the only hospitals besides the VAH. There was no Sparks Family Hospital, no outpatient facilities, no outpatient surgeries, no freestanding CAT scans, and no MRIs. Then, came the new hospital in Sparks, and health and medical care facilities proliferated all over the Truckee Meadows.

In the early days I set up my office near St. Mary's Hospital, and over the years I guess I have done sixty percent of my hospital work there. But both facilities at that time and today are quite comparable. There were occasions that one hospital would be first to purchase new equipment, but it wasn't long before the other facility would catch up. I've been quite satisfied with both hospitals over the years.

Before the advent of managed care, I admitted my patients wherever they wanted to go, but then their health care contracts specifically excluded certain facilities. It got so out of hand with all the new outpatient facilities that many of the "old timers" quit chasing facilities altogether and cut back a lot. Today I only operate at St. Mary's and Washoe. I don't go to any of the outpatient facilities, and I think it is better medicine to limit the places you admit to, as some facilities do seem to have better nursing care and some have better and more modern equipment. There may well be a higher quality of care in facilities where staffs are more familiar with individual doctor's routines.

Hospital administrators never pushed me or other ENT doctors into moneymaking ventures, and I personally never saw any of that type of commercialization. In fact, it is probably just the opposite. We have been the ones who convinced hospitals to buy equipment for new procedures that came along.

Advances in ENT

When it comes to new and innovative procedures like cochlear implants, there was a period of time when administrators were curious if there were ENT doctors in town who would be interested in starting major transplant programs.[2] There was a consensus among the ear, nose, and throat doctors that those implants should be done by trained otoneurologists in specialty centers that do hundreds of them each year, not here. It would take so much staff training and post-op treatment management that it would not be in the patient's interest if small towns and their small hospitals began doing only a few of them each year.

The need for cochlear transplants is not all that common, and I have had to refer only a handful of cases for evaluation to centers that do them. Even then, only a couple of those referred actually had the procedure done. There are other procedures, too, like acoustic neuroma removals that are so uncommon that no one in town is trained to do them and they are sent out also.[3] With those two exceptions and maybe just a few more, Reno has the expertise and the facilities for handling everything. I think we have an extremely competent and highly trained medical community.

Reconstructive Surgery

For years I did a lot of facial trauma work and a lot of reconstructive facial work, but about four or five years ago, I gave that up. There were some facial trauma panels formed and we had the option of being on them or not; at that time, I decided not to do any more facial trauma work. It wasn't that I didn't enjoy them, it was just that there were so few of them and they were quite time consuming. I also do a lot of rhinoplasty work, which is cosmetic nasal surgery, and otoplastic surgery. Another factor here is that a little rivalry between ENT doctors and plastic and reconstructive surgery doctors developed about "nose jobs" and who would do them. I've had a really good relationship with the plastic surgeons. There is very little I do that overlaps with the work of my colleagues in plastic surgery, except rhinoplasties, which I enjoy doing so much, and otoplasties for "lop" ears. We have an excellent working relationship.

ENT Procedures and Advances

This is not to say ENT doctors haven't recognized the emergence of other subspecialties that have crept into the practice of ear, nose, and throat medicine. We've had a few areas like that. When I first came to town, we did almost all the bronchoscopies for diagnosing cancer of the lung;

now, they are being done by subspecialists. ENT doctors, in fact, developed those first endoscopies. We did all bronchoscopies for the first two or three years after I arrived in town. Then, the pulmonary doctors came in and started doing them and they do a great job. We did it with rigid scopes and they do it with flexible scopes. Then, the gastroenterologists came in and started doing "scope" examinations of the GI tract.

We have a pediatric surgeon, Dr. Bill Morgan, who came to town and used scope technology for dislodging foreign bodies like peanuts from kids' lungs. So, that portion of our practice shifted to others and we began to phase it out. We still are very well trained in those procedures and we can still do some, but it is one of those areas where friendly competition was good for medicine and good for patients.

Snoring is a very common condition today and has created a lot of interest among many medical and surgical specialties. There were some studies done fifteen or twenty years ago that looked at couples and asked whether their spouses had significant snoring problems—problems like driving one or the other out of the bedroom. About seventy percent of women said their husband's had significant snoring problems, but only about thirty percent of the men said their wives were snorers. Researchers then took these same people and monitored them at night using decibel meters to measure snoring loudness. As it turned out, based on the loudness criteria they used, about fifty percent of the men had significant snoring, but forty percent of the women had snoring problems. This pointed out that women perceived their partners to have greater snoring problems than they actually did, and men underestimated the magnitude of their partner's snoring problem. This study pointed out too, that women just seem to be lighter sleepers than men. As people age, their snoring often gets worse, and studies indicate that over fifty percent of all people who snore have "sleep apnea," which can be a very serious health condition.

When it comes to any kind of surgical procedures for snoring, ENTs do the procedures, but they also work with other medical sleep specialists, like pulmonologists and neurologists.

Sleep labs have developed over the years and special breathing equipment has been created to diagnose and treat snoring and sleep apnea. The breathing device called CPAP has been a major advancement for sleep apnea, and other devices have come along for milder sleep disturbances.

Surgical procedures have also proven to be effective for snoring cures and the most recent effective surgical procedure is what we call somnoplasty, which uses radio frequency ablation by placing a probe into the palate, which diminishes snoring in ninety percent of the cases.

And so this procedure has really been a dramatic advance and it is one of the major areas of my practice today.

Just as I started practice, studies at Stanford came out on sleep apnea and researchers recognized the seriousness and frequency of this problem. Then the ear, nose, and throat specialty got interested in it back in the early 1980s.

During that time, ENTs began trimming off part of the palate and that worked well on many patients. Then the laser came along and the LAUP procedure was introduced. This is a surgical procedure in which the uvula is removed and then a procedure called "wedges of the palate," is performed—the palate is cut on each side of the uvula, and when it heals, the palate is shortened, but also stiffened. That was the procedure of choice for about ten years before the radio frequency ablation procedure was developed. I did a lot of LAUPs, probably in the neighborhood of a hundred or so up until about five years ago, when the new somnus technology came along. This relatively painless procedure was usually done in the office without major anesthesia and was more comfortable for the patients who could go back to work in a day or so, as opposed to a ten-day recovery from the previous surgical technique.

In really severe forms of sleep apnea, we do tracheotomies to open airways. These are designed to close in the daytime when patients are up and around, but they open up at night, which allows them to breathe through the tracheostomy.

There have been a lot of additional changes in my field during my career and I will mention some of the major ones. I have mentioned the use of the radio frequency ablation of the palate in the treating of snoring. Another effective use of this technology has been in straightening out the base of tongue, which has improved outcomes of cases with sleep apnea.

We use that same procedure to reduce the lining of the nose. This is a fairly new procedure that we have been doing for about five years for patients with chronic stuffiness. We use the radio frequency ablator to shrink down the lining of the nose, the area called the turbinates, and this has proven to be a real plus for the ENT practice and an advance for patients.

One of the very biggest advances in my practice has been in the treatment of sinus conditions with the introduction of sinus endoscopes. When I first started practice, if a patient had to have any kind of major sinus surgery other than in the maxillary sinuses, it was done through an outside approach because internally it was too dangerous as the sinuses are so close to the brain, the optic nerve, and carotid arteries. To do the surgery safely, we used an external approach.

The advent of the CT scan changed everything because there was a lot of sinus disease being missed on regular x-rays. The CT scan not only looks at blocked sinuses in more detail, but also gives us the advantages of seeing the cause of that blockage. Magnetic resonance imaging (MRIs) allows us to get good readings on soft tissues, but the CT scan is better for bony sinus structures.

We rarely see complicated ear infections, such as mastoiditis and meningitis, which was common in the pre-antibiotic era. I remember when I was in medical school at the University of Utah, my mentor, Dr. Dolowitz, the doctor who encouraged me to go into ENT, told me that in pre-antibiotic days, they would line kids up and do as many as seven or eight mastoidectomies every Saturday morning. Mastoiditis was rampant then, but we don't see this infection any more.

Indian Health Service

When I was in the Indian Health Service in Phoenix, we saw every complication under the sun, such as brain abscesses, meningitis, etc. Native Americans traditionally were reluctant to come in for medical care, and when they did, there was a backlog of up to nine months for treatment.

There was so much ENT work to do on the reservations. Sometimes we would hear that Native Americans had a lot of ear problems due to lack of cleanliness, sanitation, nutrition, availability of medical care, and hygiene, but in a study done by the University of Arizona comparing reservation and urban Indians, their ear problems, primarily otitis media, proved to be genetic. Studies have shown that African Americans have ear problems that also indicate a genetic link.

ENT Practice

I occasionally see elderly patients with vertigo that usually have a vascular cause due to inadequate circulation. The brain stem gets an inadequate blood supply for the balance centers. These patients get dizzy every time they stand up and have an imbalance when they walk.

There are other causes of dizziness too, probably a hundred or so different causes. One of the more common is called benign positional vertigo, which is a dizziness related to position changes. The dizziness is caused by microscopic calcium mineral deposits that build up on the small hair cells in the labyrinth area of the inner ear. Through a simple in-office technique, these deposits are repositioned through the semicircular canal; this actually works quite well to alleviate the vertigo. A lot of patients had this dizziness for years and were cured with this five-minute procedure.

Taste and smell are very important and highly complex senses. It is interesting that rarely do we find any kind of disease process that destroys the sense of taste. There are actually two different cranial nerves to the tongue that control the sense of taste, but if the sense of smell is affected, people's taste is affected even though the nerve endings for their taste sensations are intact. When things don't taste right, most patients eventually lose that sense, but it actually is a result of losing smell sensations. We see patients with anosmia, a loss of smell, which generally comes on rather acutely. We feel most of them are related to neuritis of the olfactory nerve. The olfactory nerve is probably the most delicate of all the cranial nerves and once it gets damaged, it doesn't recover.

Tobacco Use

Nevada has a higher incidence of head and neck cancer in the pharynx and larynx than the rest of the nation because of the higher incidence of smoking. We have the highest cigarette smoking consumption per capita in the United States, and we also are seeing an increased incidence of tumors in the lymph nodes of the neck. In my practice I see a lot of young people using smokeless tobacco and we try to convince them to stop that practice. I tell them, "If you chew tobacco, it's not whether you will develop cancer, it's when."

One of the most dramatic cases I've seen involved a sixteen-year-old boy from Elko who started chewing when he was age four. He developed cancer of the buccal mucosa and it was hard for me to believe his uncle introduced him to tobacco.

People who smoke cigarettes and don't drink alcohol have a higher incidence of oral cancer than non-smokers, but if you add alcohol to the equation, cancer incidence goes up many fold. I think it's because the alcohol wipes off the protective mucous coating of the throat so the tobacco has more irritating potential. It's a lethal combination.

Body Piercing

A patient occasionally asks me about complications of their kid piercing their tongues, but I have only seen one untoward reaction. It was a young lady who developed an infection and a localized abscess where tongue tissue grew around the stud. I had to take it out surgically. That is the only complication I have seen. Every now and then I treat nasal obstruction caused by nose piercing, which can be serious, but I have only seen a few earlobe piercings that got infected.

Organized Medicine

I became interested and involved in organized medicine at the Washoe County Medical Society level when I first moved to town and stayed active for about fifteen years. I was a county society representative to the Nevada State Medical Association House of Delegates for many of those years, but the last eight or nine years I have cut back on that involvement to spend more time at home. I am currently chairman of the ENT department at Washoe Medical Center and there is something going on almost every night. Serving on committees and being active in political activities is very time consuming, and can be quite disruptive to a practice.

Managed Care

Managed care, however, has changed medicine dramatically and requires almost continuous watching by practicing physicians. It has taken a lot of fun out of medicine in spite of the seemingly good intentions of trying to reduce medical costs. Actually, managed care has increased costs because of the extra tier of administrative expense that business is imposing. Doctors, hospitals, and pharmacies are making less than they did in 1975 and health insurance premiums keep going up. The question is, "Where is the money going?" Even after you factor in the huge cost of improved technology and drugs and the increased number of services offered, managed care is still the culprit.

One of the things so disappointing to me is that quality of care does not enter into the bottom line with managed care organizations. I would never have thought that would happen, even ten years ago. Those companies look for the providers who will sign the least expensive contracts without regard to the skills, abilities, and reputation of those providers. That is very disappointing! Those of us who have been around a long time still have good practices, realizing that patients are really shuffled around by managed care plans. No longer do they have the choice of physician or hospital.

Another area that has been of great concern to me is managed care making medical decisions on which drugs and tests to order and use, and which procedures to perform. This adds another whole level of paperwork in doctor's offices to comply with prior authorizations and such, and to do the accounting necessary to assure payments. The first ten years I was in practice, I would run my office with two staff members; I'm no busier now than I was then, but now there are five staff members. Overhead goes up and reimbursements go down. Patients start wondering why physicians recommend a certain procedure or test that is not approved by their insurance company, and they begin to wonder why a doctor's fee has been cut in half by their insurance company. These things create a rift in the physician-patient relationship.

I am one of the doctors in northern Nevada that will take all patients regardless of their insurance, or source of payment. I was pleased to see Washoe County Medical Society sponsor the Health Access Washoe County Clinic, and I take every patient HAWC sends over to me. I also see patients St. Mary's Hospital sends me from their Sun Valley and Neil Road clinics.

It is discouraging to hear that less than half of the ENT doctors in town will see Medicare patients. They get funneled into my office. If each doctor would take his or her share, then it wouldn't be so overwhelming. I feel some obligation to provide my services to seniors as I approach Medicare age myself, and I sometimes wonder who will take care of me when I'm on Medicare.

I have two daughters and a son and they have all grown up here and done well. My middle daughter is in her chief year of otolaryngology at Northwestern in Chicago and elected to go into medicine and into my specialty all on her own; however, I did encourage her a little. From age eleven, Courtney told me she wanted to be a doctor and she has never varied from that course. I think she appreciates that it is the premier specialty because ENTs have such an interesting surgical and office practice.

My practice, raising my family, and my life in Reno have really been great. I have always enjoyed medicine and will continue to do that; I don't look forward to the idea of retirement at all.

Notes
[1] Dr. Olin Moulton was born in Maine in 1908 and licensed in Nevada in 1936. Dr. John Brophy was born in North Dakota in 1926 and licensed in Nevada in 1956.

[2] A cochlear implant is a substitute for the middle ear that is necessary for hearing.

[3] Acoustic neuroma is a benign tumor on the acoustic nerve near the brain. It is considered brain surgery.

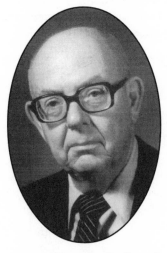
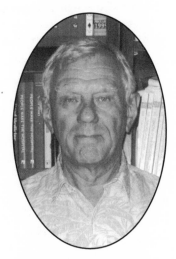

Dr. Owen C. Bolstad   Dr. Anton P. Sohn

11: Drs. Owen C. Bolstad and Anton Sohn, Pathology[1]

Dr. Owen C. Bolstad

Education

Owen C. Bolstad was born March 8, 1921, and lived in a small Minnesota farming community the first twenty years of his life. His school was adjourned for a week each year so the students could help on the farm. Most of his schoolmates were destined to remain in the farming community, but Owen and his best friend, Neil Osmundson, saw college as their way to a bigger world. Unfortunately, Appleton High School did not offer college prep courses, so Owen and Neil had to request that physics be added to the curriculum; and it didn't hurt that Owen's father, a veterinarian, was on the school board. During their junior year of high school, Owen and Neil joined the Minnesota National Guard, in which they remained active for four years. After high school, there was anticipation in the air as the economy improved, but Europe teetered on the brink with war on the horizon. It was the best of times for Owen and the worse of times for world peace. Owen's friend, Bill Kaufman recalled:

> In the time between Owen's graduation from high
> school [1939] and the federalizing of the Guard [1941], he

attended the local University of Minnesota Extension taking basic college courses. He also worked at Carl Miller's Grocery, driving the delivery truck (groceries were delivered throughout the town then) and stocking shelves, etc.

He owned a canoe and a Model A Ford coupe—both the envy of many. I don't think he used the canoe to fish, but we hunted ducks and pheasants. I had a Cushman Autoglide motor scooter—a pretty decent piece of machinery, and Neil and Owen would steal it regularly and take a ride while I was in school—something of a game to them, but very irritating to me. Another activity was a sort of "car tag," up and down alleys—usually late at night. Owen in his Model A, Neil in his '34 Ford sedan, and a young lady, Betty Hanson, (who later was a bomber ferry pilot in the Wasps) was a worthy competitor in her Model A sedan. The police were either quite understanding or inept.

Neil owned a Snipe sailboat and a spring ritual was painting it, putting a new anchorage into Lac qui Parle, and putting the boat in the water. On Sunday and in the evenings sailing was a favorite summer activity. The fall ritual was putting the boat up for the winter.

Life in the small town was not terribly exciting— probably why so many of us left. This is how I remember it. It was a long time ago.[1]

U.S. Army and World War II

After the government activated the Guard in 1941, the unit took basic training in Louisiana. Owen, who was in the infantry, saw hostile action in North Africa and Italy. Discharged from the army, he and Neil enrolled at the University of Minnesota on the GI bill and studied engineering. Unable to decide on a future specialty in engineering, Owen took a battery of aptitude tests and was informed that his skills and interest were better suited to a career in medicine. After studying premed at the University of Minnesota and enrolling in medical school, Owen met his future wife, Katie. They married in 1949 between his second and third year of medical school.

Internship, General Practice, and Pathology

The family moved to Duluth for Owen's internship, and then he set up practice in Little Falls, Minnesota, where he practiced for ten years. Katie remembers the good times in Little Falls when the growing family rode their bikes on family excursions; however, two weeks before Christmas, Dr. Bolstad came home and said he was quitting practice and going to take a residency in pathology. Katie was devastated when told they were leaving. The family stayed in Little Falls during the first year of residency while Owen lived in St. Paul. It was uncomfortable for Katie, because Owen was well liked by his patients, and they let her know that they were unhappy with his choice.

During the general practice years, the family always headed west to the mountains for vacation; therefore, it was only natural that Dr. Bolstad would come to the West to practice pathology. When the decision was made to come to Reno, the chief of pathology at the Veterans Administration Hospital in St. Paul, like so many who have a misconception of life in Reno, asked if there were any churches in Reno.

Pathology in Reno (Bolstad)

History of Pathology in Reno
When Dr. Bolstad came to Reno in 1966, there were two groups of pathologists.[2] The oldest group, Dr. V. A. Salvadorini's, was known as Laboratory Medicine Consultants (LMC), and Dr. Schieve headed the other group, Western Clinical Laboratories (WCL). Dr. Salvadorini came to Reno in 1951 and with Dr. Lawrence Parsons, formed an outpatient laboratory, which eventually became LMC.

Dr. Parsons came to Reno in 1933 and worked with Dr. Alice Thompson, a Nevada native who directed the State Hygienic Laboratory, now the State Public Health Laboratory. In 1934 she became the consulting pathologist at Washoe General Hospital (now Washoe Medical Center), and Dr. Parsons eventually went to Saint Mary's Hospital (SMH) to head its laboratory. Washoe General Hospital did not have funds to start a clinical laboratory, so all chemistry and bacteriology tests were sent to the State Hygienic Laboratory.

The Parsons and Salvadorini laboratory grew and by 1964, LMC had contracts at Washoe Medical Center (WMC) and Saint Mary's Hospital, as well as the Reno Veterans Administration Hospital.[3] Dr. Don Schieve's laboratory business was also growing. Dr. Bolstad recalled:

> Dr. Don Schieve arrived on the scene in 1964. He
> began to develop contacts with a lot of the younger doctors
> in town, who rather resented the monopoly enjoyed by the

Salvadorini group and welcomed a competitor. Don began by buying out a local bioanalyst, Everett Warren, who had a contract with Carson-Tahoe Hospital. Don loved to fly and offered to provide autopsy service to many of the outlying counties in Nevada and California. Contracts with Weimar Sanitarium, Barton Memorial, Plumas District, Bishop, Elko General, Pershing General, and Carlin Hospitals became more than he could handle, so he took me on as a partner in 1966.

Don loved to fly and was a good, competent pilot. When I first came to town, the lab had a Cessna 175—an oddball aircraft with a geared propeller. The plane had a distressing habit of overheating the back cylinders on prolonged climb-out. This resulted in high repair and maintenance costs. We then bought a Beechcraft VTC 35 Bonanza, a real deluxe bird that cruised at nearly 190 knots per hour. Our practice thrived, and in 1971 we began construction of a large laboratory facility at 888 Willow Street. The proximity of competition so close to Washoe Medical Center caused some anxiety with LMC.

Dr. Schieve was aggressive in approaching hospitals serviced by LMC, while the Salvadorini group did everything possible to keep Schieve's group out of Reno hospitals. This practice continued until 1971, when coincidental with construction of a central laboratory at 888 Willow Street facility by WCL, the first giant step in automation of chemistry tests in Reno took place and forced the groups to work together. At that time LMC had a building on Aiken Street, one block from Washoe Medical Center, where Dr. James Decker worked with the Robot Chemist, an automated chemistry analyzer. Decker and medical technologist David Hahn had problems with the reliability of the Robot Chemist, and it was eventually abandoned. The LMC group voted four to one to approach WCL to jointly buy an Autoanalyzer that would do twelve chemistry tests on one sample of blood.[4]

Drs. Decker and Schieve knew each other from playing golf at the Hidden Valley Country Club where Decker brought up the idea of each providing one half of the $100,000 to buy the equipment. The members of WCL were interested, but only if the two groups merged and all of the partners became equal. As Dr. Bill Keenan, one of the WCL partners so eloquently put it, "There would be no sacred cows."

Dr. Anton P. Sohn

Education

I was born on October 1, 1935, in Indianapolis, Indiana of middle class, deeply religious parents. My mother, who was a public health nurse before I was born, and my uncle, who was dentist were the strong medical influences in my life. On the other hand, my father, Anton Peter, who only finished the sixth grade, was adamant that all of the Sohn kids would get a college education. As a result of strong family influence, all four of the Sohn siblings graduated from college.

My interest was in math, art, and architectural drafting. During two years of studying architecture at the University of Cincinnati, I was influenced by my premed friends and decided to take biology in summer school. I, not only, found science more interesting than architecture, but also found medicine more challenging. After graduation from the Indiana University School of Medicine in 1961, I was lured by the open spaces and mountains of the West and went to San Francisco General Hospital to do an internship. Unfortunately, my father died that year and after my internship, I returned to Indianapolis and did general practice for six months. The best part of that six months was meeting Arlene, who became my wife.

Training in Forensic and General Pathology

During general practice in Indiana, I decided that pathology appealed to my interest in studying diseases. Furthermore, I had an interest in forensic pathology and solving the related puzzles of crime. I talked to Dr. Ed Smith, the chairman of pathology at Indiana University and he suggested that I contact Dr. Charles Larson, who was a leading forensic pathologist and headed the pathology program in Tacoma, Washington. After Arlene and I married in 1963, we bundled up all of our belongings in a U-hall trailer and headed west. Arlene and I had a glorious time in Tacoma and saw all parts of the state, hiking, camping, fishing, and climbing mountains. At the end of our third year in the Northwest, we had our first son, Anton Phillip, and the army came knocking the day he was born.

The U.S. Army and Vietnam

After I was drafted, I was stationed at Ford Ord in Monterey, California. While there we hiked the Sierra Nevada and explored the Monterey peninsula. In the fall 1966, we got the call that would lead us to Reno. Dr. Ron Cudek, a classmate from med school, called and invited us to Reno for Thanksgiving. That winter another order from the U.S. Government assigned me to Vietnam. Since I was the only trained forensic pathologist in that country, I went to Saigon to head up the anatomical and forensic pathology division. This was an interesting year as my division investigated all deaths unrelated to hostile action and crimes committed by U.S. servicemen in South Vietnam. Maybe some day I will write about my experiences there; however, during that year, I got a letter from Dr. Cudek stating that there were openings in Reno for two pathologists.

After I was discharged from the army, Arlene and I traveled to Reno and interviewed with both pathology groups: each was recruiting for a new pathologist. We accepted employment with Dr. Salvadorini's group, Laboratory Medicine Consultants, because it had a stable practice and covered the pathology service at all of the Reno hospitals.

Pathology in Reno (Sohn)

Move to Reno

We moved to Reno in June 1968, and knew we had found the perfect place to practice medicine and raise our family. Our last two children, Eric and Kristin, were born in Reno. And I was actually getting paid to do something that I loved to do. After three years with LMC, a merger would make the first of many changes in my practice.

A Merger and a Centralized Lab

After the merger, the new group of twelve pathologists eventually grew to twenty-four members. The centralized laboratory at 888 Willow opened on September 18, 1972 and provided a wider range of tests and a decreased cost when analyzed in batches.[5] This reference laboratory could also do complex and infrequently ordered tests by centralizing the specimens from all hospitals and outlying labs in one facility.

Surgical Pathology

In addition to clinical tests, the LMC/WCL group provided surgical specimen evaluation at the central facility and visited rural hospitals to perform frozen section diagnosis in the operation room. These visits to rural hospitals were coordinated with medical staff meetings and scheduled surgery that required a pathologist for frozen section diagnosis. The pathologist transported a microtome that connected to a canister of carbon dioxide to quick-freeze tissue.[6] A small piece of a tumor excised during surgery, for example a breast biopsy, was cut into thin slices. The sliver of tissue was placed on a glass slide, stained with a methylene blue solution, and examined under a microscope. Many times the stained tissue was poorly cut and poorly stained making interpretation difficult. This forced the pathologist to rely on his gross examination of the tumor to determine whether it was malignant.

In the 1960s the cryostat replaced the cumbersome microtome. The cryostat, one of which was kept on each hospital's premises, is an insulated container that houses the microtome in a subfreezing environment. This advance made the frozen section diagnosis more reliable for the surgeon, who used the information to decide on the proper operation.

A Split in the Merger

Dr. Bolstad continued with his insight into the dynamics of interpersonal relationships of the pathology partners:

> The merged group continued to expand, acquiring hospitals in Roseville and Auburn, California. In 1985 the group assumed responsibility for teaching pathology at the University of Nevada School of Medicine. By that time the twenty-four pathologists began to have internal problems. It became unwieldy to administer and maintain quality control. There were differences in the philosophy of practice and tensions grew due to unequal workloads. Eventually these problems resulted in the dissolution of the merged group in 1988 when Washoe Health Systems, the parent organization of WMC, bought out eighteen of the partners and fifty-one percent of the laboratory. In 1992 Washoe Health Systems forced the sale of the laboratory to Allied Laboratories, Inc., a huge national corporation.

The Status of Pathology in 1950

What was the practice of pathology and clinical laboratory medicine, known as clinical pathology, like before the merger? Many of the tests in the 1950s had been used for fifty years, and there was little advancement until after World War II. Probably the most important change during the war was the organization of a blood banking system, which provided whole blood and plasma to wounded servicemen. Dr. Charles Drew, an African-American and the first director of the American Red Cross Blood Bank, devised a system of separating plasma from red blood cells which prolonged the life of blood components. Plasma could be frozen and stored for long periods and shipped to the battlefront while red blood cells had a much shorter shelf life and had to be used within weeks.

After the war, pathologists returned home and organized blood banks in their communities, and a nationwide system sprang up providing blood products for emergencies. (See the blood bank paragraph.)

In many ways the laboratory of fifty years ago was vastly different from the modern laboratory, but its basic function was the same and its organization by departments has not changed greatly. The basic components of a laboratory are hematology, coagulation, urinalysis, chemistry, serology (now called immunology), blood banking, toxicology, cytology, tissue pathology, and microbiology. To this array of specialties, a bioterrorism section has been added to the public health laboratory and DNA technology was added to the regional reference laboratory.

Advances in Pathology and the Clinical Laboratory

During the past fifty years, the clinical laboratory has become more specialized and a greater number of tests are offered. Just as important, many of today's tests have greater sensitivity and specificity, allowing diseases to be detected earlier and with more certainty. In addition many assays are now available in a diagnostic kit with simple outlined steps, thereby decreasing the complexity for workers.

On another front, reimbursement for patient testing by government and insurance companies has changed the industry by capping reimbursement. The regional private laboratory in Nevada has become a thing of the past. Two large multibillion-dollar corporations bought up Nevada's two regional private laboratories, one of which was Sierra Nevada Laboratories. Outpatient laboratory services in Nevada are now part of a nationwide industry where market pressure, competition, and stockholders emphasize profit, many times making it more important than patient care.

In the following paragraphs I will delineate what I consider to be the most important advancements in the clinical laboratory in Reno since the 1950s. The American Society of Clinical Pathology (ASCP) is the scientific arm of practicing pathologists and leads the way in disseminating the latest advances in the clinical laboratory. In the 1970s and 1980s all Reno pathologists belonged to the ASCP. It held regional and annual meetings with seminars and hands-on laboratories to demonstrate the latest scientific techniques to its members. I have attended these meetings to learn the latest in laboratory medicine, but ninety-nine percent of the time the advances they demonstrated were already in use in Reno. Since the 1950s laboratory medicine in Reno was always on the cutting edge, and the tests necessary for patient care were available here at the same time they were provided at major medical centers in the rest of the country. Only esoteric tests that were done at research centers had to be sent out of state.

In the 1950s statistical quality control became a requirement for the modern clinical laboratory, and by the late 1960s, handheld computers were used in all Reno laboratories. By 1980, larger computers were used to calculate quality control and to order, report, store, and analyze tests. On June 21, 1982, WMC offered the first laboratory-wide computer with reports that provided instant results to the patient's chart on the ward. It also made ordering of tests quicker and easier for the nurse, but it created problems with the growing pieces of paper for the patient's chart.

To convince the board of trustees of the value of spending $800,000 for the computer, the laboratory did a study. We assumed there was a significant number of tests done by the laboratory that were not charged because the hand-produced charge slips were difficult to control. In the study one hundred consecutive patient charts were reviewed for tests ordered, tests done, and tests charged. The review found that there were four percent undercharges and four percent overcharges. The financial significance was that the new computer caused zero impact on the bottom line of the hospital. Another argument for computerization was that personnel would be eliminated. This assumption was found to be false. It was also argued that fewer office workers would be needed in the future, but no retrospective study has been done to verify this assertion.

In the early 1980s simple prepackaged reagents using specific antibodies directed against a specific substance to be analyzed became available in Reno laboratories. This advance led to home pregnancy, drug, and cholesterol testing by patients. Twenty years later high-precision and high-stability analyzers were introduced in Reno, leading to increased precision of results.

The following described advances in the clinical laboratory are just a few of the thousands of new tests and changes in techniques that occurred during the last half of the twentieth century. The changes in hematology led the way in the clinical laboratory, and automation of the blood cell count was the first step.

After development of the automated white and red cell counter, scientists in the early 1970s at the Los Alamos National Laboratories developed a flow cytometer that used a laser beam to count specific cells that scattered the light in a characteristic diagnostic manner. This technique is useful as an aid to diagnose and treat cancer, AIDS-associated disease, and anemia. The blood clotting lab, a subsection of hematology, also saw advances.

The history of clotting studies dates to before 1910 when it was noted that a white horse hair, when drawn through blood that was beginning to clot, turned red when the early clot on the hair trapped red blood cells. The first major step in clotting studies came in 1912 when Dr. Roger Lee and famed cardiologist Paul Dudley White developed the Lee-White clotting test to monitor patients treated with heparin after a heart attack. A stopwatch was used to record when blood clotted in a test tube. The Lee-White clotting time was replaced in the 1950s at WMC and SMH when the activated partial thromboplastin time (aPTT) test was introduced. The aPTT test measures, in seconds, how long it takes for a clot to form when the plasma is mixed with an activator and calcium. This procedure moved the test from the bedside to the laboratory, where the test was more controlled and took less labor. Another important test in the hematology section is the urinalysis.

The lowly urinalysis has always been a mainstay in the clinical laboratory. It requires the specimen to be centrifuged and the sediment to be microscopically evaluated. Under the microscope, red and white blood cells are identified and counted. In the 1960s, the Ames Corporation developed the dipstick test, whereby a paper slip impregnated with a chemical is dipped in the urine and the intensity of the color reaction indicates the level of the substance tested. As a result of this new technology, personnel with little training could do the test in any doctor's office. Matching strides with advances in hematology was the chemistry section.

Maybe the greatest strides in the clinical laboratory were in the chemistry section, where automation was used to increase the efficiency and lower the cost. The automated chemistry analyzer, the Autoanalyzer, was the first with automation of the blood glucose, which became available in Reno in the 1960s. Aside from automation, another important advance was the radioimmunoassay (RIA) based on radioactive material that can be attached to antibodies and then counted using a gamma counter. This test was more sensitive and detected minute amounts of substances that previous assays could not detect.[7] The procedure opened the way for the routine testing of diabetes, thyroid diseases, reproductive disorders, hypertension, and other diseases, and it was not influenced by interfering medication. The RIA was first offered in Reno in March 1973, and the laboratory diagnosis of endocrine disease was solved.

The diagnosis of endocrine diseases has always been an enigma for physicians. Before the RIA, thyroid function was evaluated by a blood test that was influenced by many drugs and conditions other than thyroid disease. The physician had to rely on clinical judgement to make the diagnosis.[8] On July 15, 1976, the chemistry panel at WMC was increased from fourteen to seventeen tests for $16.50 (no additional cost to the patient). At the same time WCL joined with Sacramento Clinical Laboratory to offer a panel of twenty-two chemistry tests for sixteen dollars. In addition to chemistry, blood banking saw changes.

Blood banking in Reno dates to 1947 when Pathologist Lawrence Parsons agreed to supervise the blood band at WMC. However the supply of banked blood was not a priority until 1955 when doctors recommended that full obstetrical services and a staffed recovery room be added to Washoe Medical Center. Dr. Salvadorini, who was then chief of the laboratory, took the problem of an inadequate supply of blood to the Washoe County Medical Society. A committee of the Society approached Southwest Blood Bank of Phoenix, which signed a contract in 1956 to become WMC's blood bank. The hospital made available a World War II Quonset hut on its campus to house the blood drawing and storage facility. The Southwest Blood Bank still supplies blood to all of Nevada. The advances in blood banking saved lives and decreased morbidity in diseases such as hemophilia, but the development of gyn cytology saved the lives of thousands of women from the slow death of cancer of the uterine cervix.

In 1943 George Papanicolaou and Herbert Traut published an article demonstrating that uterine cancer could be diagnosed on a cervical smear, the Pap smear. The Pap smear became a routine test in Reno laboratories in the early 1960s. Study of the Pap smear led to the discovery in 1970 that cancer of the cervix is caused by the human papilloma virus (HPV). Changes of HPV can be identified microscopically on the Pap smear or by a lab test on the liquid suspended cells. When detected early, cancer of the cervix can be prevented.

The last area in the modern clinical laboratory to be discussed is the cytogenetics laboratory and the DNA laboratory. The first cytogenetics laboratory in Nevada was created in 1988 through a joint venture agreement between the University of Nevada School of Medicine and Sierra Nevada Laboratories. Amniotic fluid cells from pregnant women were cultured and examined under the microscope. This allowed the prenatal diagnosis of congenital disorders so that the doctor could better treat the newborn infant.

Dr. Steve St. Jeor started the first DNA laboratory in Nevada at the University of Nevada School of Medicine in 1991. The lab utilizes a technique that takes a small fragment of deoxyribonucleic acid (DNA) and multiplies it by the polymerase chain reaction (PCR) method that was devised by scientists in 1983. The DNA test is 99.999+ percent accurate in establishing or excluding paternity by comparing an individual's genetic makeup to family members.

Like all branches of medicine, the clinical laboratory has seen remarkable advances. Advances have come from space exploration laboratories, the computer industry, and technology unrelated to medicine, but the application of these fields has been driven by professionals within the clinical laboratory. No matter what changes in techniques, equipment, or reagents will come in the twenty-first century, the role of the laboratory in patient diagnosis and treatment will continue.

Looking Back

I think I am the luckiest pathologist in Reno. I have been able to start a new and more exciting career every five or six years. First, I was a staff pathologist at Washoe Medical Center and the consulting pathologist at the VAH. During that time I pursued forensic pathology in the Washoe County Coroner's office and northern Nevada. When Dr. Salvadorini retired, I became chief of the WMC's lab. Then, I began a career in medical politics: chief of staff at WMC, president of Washoe County Medical Society, Nevada State Medical Association, and Reno surgical Society. A pathologist with predominately a desk job is ideally suited for administrative functions and serving the medical profession in addition to serving patients.

In 1985 I became chairman of the department of pathology at the School of Medicine, which led to another career: medical historian. The Nevada State Medical Association sparked my interest in the history of medicine when I met older doctors from around the state, who told stories of medicine in the old days. I saw a need to preserve the history of medicine in Nevada, and the School of Medicine gave me the means to accomplish that goal. As a result of this vision, Dr. Bolstad and I started the history of medicine program. In 2002 we dedicated a history of medicine library and museum at the School in Reno, part of which is dedicated to Dr. Bolstad's memory. My career is now dedicated to researching and recording Nevada's history of health sciences.

Notes

[1] Dr. Owen Bolstad started this chapter during the winter of 2001-2, but he died on February 20, 2002, before it was finished. Dr. Bolstad's widow, Katie, supplied information about the pre-Reno years; his boyhood friend, Bill Kaufman, added information about the two years after high school; and Dr. Anton Sohn finished the Reno years.

[2] Email from Bill Kaufman November 19, 2002.

[3] The seven members of Laboratory Medicine Consultants were Drs. John W. Callister, James W. Decker, Thomas E. Hall, Frederick A. Laubscher, Vasco A. Salvadorini, Anton P. Sohn, and James M. Tenney. The five members of Western Clinical Laboratories were Drs. Owen C. Bolstad, Theodore G. Goldfarb, William J. Keenan, Donald R. Schieve, and D. Jack Stouder.

[4] The first known pathologist in Reno was Dr. Lawrence Parsons. The first full-time pathologist at Washoe Medical Center (WMC) was Dr. Alice Thompson, who was also the first woman physician at WMC. Dr. Salvadorini was recruited by Dr. William Mack to come to WMC. Dr. Salvadorini was instrumental in forming WMC's first twenty-four hour clinical laboratory.

[5] The first single channel Autoanalyzer was developed by Technicon Corporation in the 1950s, and as the technology evolved, multiple fully automated channels became available. The twenty-two-channel analyzer cost $239,000 in 1977.

[6] When the central facility at 888 Willow opened in 1972, the twelve automated tests cost the patient $10.

[7] The microtome consists of a metal block where the tissue is frozen and a knife cuts a thin sliver of tissue less than one cell in thickness.

[8] Dr. Solomon A. Berson and researcher Rosalyn Yalow developed the RIA in the 1950s. In 1977 Yalow received the Nobel Prize for this achievement.

[9] Over twenty drugs and various medical conditions are recording in the medical literature as altering the PBI and T4 test for thyroid function.

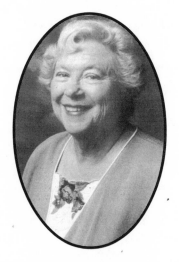

12: Dr. Francine Mannix, Pediatrics

Dr. Francine Mannix

Early Life

I was born September 11, 1935, in Hollywood, California, and when I was six years old, my mother divorced my father and took my sister and me back to her home in Montana to live with my grandmother. She remarried and we lived on a cattle ranch. I remember going to a typical one-room schoolhouse with grades six through eight, located about three miles from my home. One winter my teacher lived with us and frequently we had to get to school by sleigh. I started middle school and high school in Deer Lodge, Montana, where the old territorial prison, built back in the 1880s, was located. A new prison is there now.

The first two years of high school I was interested in becoming a chemical engineer, and I took a lot of Latin classes because I understood I had to have some background in Latin. When I was starting my third year, I moved back to California to live with my father and his wife. I finished high school in Glendale. Meanwhile, my mother divorced and remarried a professor of agriculture at the University of Nevada and I joined her in Reno in 1953.

My first job in Reno was as an assistant to banker Jordan Crouch at the headquarters office of the First National Bank of Nevada.[1] I worked there during my first year of college and during my second year, I got a job as a receptionist at KZTV and became secretary to station owner, Donald W. Reynolds. The station was renamed KOLO TV and Mr. Reynolds was honored later by having the University's School of Journalism named after him.[2]

Since I was certain I wanted to be a chemical engineer in high school, I began chemistry studies, but got sidetracked by my stepfather who encouraged me to consider a medical career. My schooling was interrupted by my various jobs as a secretary and a switchboard operator, thus causing me to drop out one semester, which delayed my graduating from college by one year.

Medical School

I applied to medical school and sent applications to Cornell, Yale, Utah, UGLA, and USC, and I still remember having to come up with $50 for each application—that was a lot of money back then.

I had an interview in Salt Lake City and was delayed in getting admitted, but I don't think I had much chance of being picked anyway. The committee only accepted four out-of-state students each year, and the interview team consisted of a room full of psychiatrists who never smiled. Maybe their frowns were a result of my being an hour late for the interview.

At USC I interviewed by Dr. Helen Martin, also called the "Grand Old Dame of Diabetes." Months went by and I heard nothing. I was working at KOLO then and was offered the job of program manager. I thought long and hard about accepting it, but I still wanted to go to medical school.

I was encouraged to talk with Reno surgeon, Wesley W. Hall, M.D., who was on the board of trustees of the American Medical Association, to see if he would use his influence to help me get accepted at his alma mater, Tulane University, but then I got the letter of acceptance from USC medical school.[3]

My dad and his wife were living in southern California when I returned to go to school. There was talk of my living with them, but I spent the first year on campus in student housing as everything pretty much was on the USC campus. They didn't have the medical school housing like they have now, so there was a lot of driving involved.

After my first year in med school, I returned to Reno and got a summer job working for Dr. William Keezer, a general practitioner in Carson City.[4] I would drive back and forth. As a first year med student, he allowed me to do a lot of interesting medical things and I became his nurse of sorts. It's funny what comes to mind today about working there. We sterilized syringes in his office by boiling them in vinegar water. Interesting! The first injection I ever gave, a penicillin shot, was to an inmate at the women's prison. That poor thing! One time Dr. Keezer left me completely in charge of his office and I had to take care of an injured dog. I think I did some suturing on the dog.

On a number of occasions, I would no sooner get home than the doctor would call saying, "I'm going to do an autopsy. Do you want to come back?" I was very eager at that time and headed right back to Carson to watch the autopsy, which was done at a mortuary across from the Capitol. He took an interest in me, encouraged me, and influenced me quite a lot.

I had gone to medical school wanting to be a brain surgeon or a psychiatrist, but the first time I observed a well-known USC pediatrician handle an infant, my mind was made up: I would go into pediatrics. Besides, the psychiatrists I dealt with seemed kind of nutsy. I have no idea where my original thoughts of becoming a brain surgeon went.

A Job in Medical School

My mother had been a dealer at the Nevada Club in Reno the entire time I was in school and had worked there for a total of thirteen years. She dealt craps, roulette, and twenty-one. One summer I worked in the Nevada Club as a change carrier but only lasted a few days as the change was entirely too heavy for me. I went to the owner, Mr. Lincoln Fitzgerald, saying, "You know, my mother has taught me to deal twenty-one on the ironing board in our basement, would you please let me try to be a twenty-one dealer?" He consented and I dealt double-deck black jack on the graveyard shift and later graduated to single-deck.

Mom used to tell me about Lavere Redfield, the reclusive Reno millionaire, who would come into the club looking very much like a farmer, a hayseed. He would go into the office and get chips and she didn't know if they were $1 chips or $10,000 chips.

Internship and Residency

I think my training at USC was excellent, because students were allowed to do so many things that would not be permitted at other places. Six of my med school friends and I went to Fresno for our internship, and we got a few laughs when we saw surgical residents from Stanford who got so little hands-on training that all they were allowed to do in surgery was handle retractors.

After a year at Fresno, it was off to Kowakilani Children's Hospital in Hawaii for my pediatrics residency. My mother became quite ill, so I headed back to Los Angeles for my second year of residency to be closer to her. I worked in the fairly new intensive care units for premature infants at the county hospital, which was just beginning at that time. They were also just starting to do blood gases.

It was an interesting time for pediatrics back in 1964 and 1965 when the measles vaccine came out and oral polio drugs were being administered. I remember seeing a lot of meningitis and the incidence of diphtheria was high. Surprisingly there was also a fair amount of tetanus in the area, but there were some pretty good drugs available for infectious diseases, such as Ampicillin and Chloromycetin.

Reno Pediatrics

Early Pediatricians

I finished my pediatric residency training in late 1965 and returned to Reno to set up my practice in January 1966 at 890 Mill Street. I went in with a pediatrician named Dr. Carl Zigenhorn. He had been practicing with Dr. Roland Stahr who had just retired.[5] I believe there was one other pediatric group in town composed of Drs. John Palmer, William Pasutti, John Scott, and Emanuel "Bud" Berger.[6] Dr. Scott told me of his experiences he had working with the Crippled Children's Service on the Indian reservations. He found all these dislocated hips because of the way women carried their children. They put them on carrying boards rather than carrying them on their hips, so the hips were not ever in the socket correctly. This created a chronic problem in the Native American population in Nevada. Drs. Scott and Berger were in town during the polio epidemic and operated all the iron lung machines in town, which were later stored in the basement at Washoe Medical Center.

Medicine in Reno was state-of-the-art, and my stepfather spoke very highly of several doctors in the area: Drs. Louie Lombardi, Ken Maclean, Bob Crosby, Bill O'Brien, and many others.[77]

Dr. Maclean was a member of and chief spokesman for the Nevada Board of Medical Examiners, and every doctor who came to the state had to go before his group. When I appeared before the board for licensure, I can still remember the question Dr. Maclean asked me, which was, "What about an umbilical hernia?" I said, "Well, we don't get too excited about them until they are five or six years," and that seemed to be the right answer.

Pediatric Diseases

My associate, Dr. Zigenhorn, who was a man in his early fifties, died shortly after I joined him. One of my first patients, a very sick four-year old girl, turned out to be a nightmare right from the start. I had admitted her with a very high temperature (105 degrees) and she was later diagnosed with meningococcal meningitis and subsequently became comatose and lost her limbs as a result of gangrene. I felt like I had a black cloud over my head. She was a remarkable little Mexican girl and her treatment challenged me to the maximum as she was in the hospital from April to September that year. She later received prosthetic arms, but prosthetic legs would not work for her. I followed her for years and found out she went on to study psychology at Truckee Meadows Community College and later got married.

I was always concerned about the high incidence of cancer in this area and thought the atomic testing done in the central part of the state had something to do with the rare cancers we see. Several movie stars, who were working on location in Nevada and Utah years ago, came down with cancers: John Wayne, Susan Hayward, and Agnes Moorhead, just to name a few, indicating something was going on here. I've always thought there is entirely too much cancer in children in this area also.

In addition to polio and its subsequent massive immunization programs, children in Reno were being skin tested for tuberculosis in all the schools. I recall one family in which the father was a dealer at the Nevada Club and all the adults in his family must have had active TB. When the kids tested positive, I referred them to the Weimar Tuberculosis Center for treatment. I was a dealer at the Nevada Club earlier, and we all had to have mini-chest x-rays; and if we handled food, we had to have skin tests in order to get health cards.

I spent most of my first years primarily at Washoe Medical Center primarily because at that time St. Mary's did not have an emergency room. In fact, I had very little to do with Saints because there were no ER facilities. Very sick patients with very rare diseases and illnesses would be sent to Sacramento, Oakland, or to UCSF. It is interesting that we called the place where we treated sick babies the "Preemie Nursery" and staffed it on a volunteer basis. Today it has evolved and is called the "Neonatal Intensive Care Unit" with full-time specialists and high tech equipment.

Pediatric Specialization

Pediatricians began to sub-specialize and got extra training as neonatal intensivists, hematologists, pulmonologists, cardiologists, surgeons, and other neonatal sub-specialties. Over the years Reno had a couple of pediatric surgeons that came and went, but we have an excellent one now in Dr. Bill Morgan, a very skilled and humane man.

The medical school was in the early planning stages when I came to town, but I never really got involved. I was just too busy. I have realized pediatricians do not, as a rule, join lots of clubs, organizations, and movements and generally don't socialize with each other very much. That's just the way we are. One time, many years ago, area pediatricians formed a journal club, and I think we had one or two Academy of Pediatrics meetings in which one of the doctors from Las Vegas would come up and present papers. Some of us, because we were so busy working nights and days, had to periodically close our practices to new patients. I had to do that after the first ten years of my work in town.

Organized Medicine

I have always been a member of the county medical society, state association, and the AMA. For a while, I belonged to the American Medical Women's Association, which wasn't very active, but it is more active now with more women physicians practicing here. I put time in the Nevada Chapter of the American Heart Association as president and worked with children at the state mental hospital at Lake's Crossing. Frequently I would work at the Crippled Children's Clinic, and I served on the Board of Nevada Self-Help. I guess I have been fairly active in medical organizations over the years.

My Reno Practice

Reno was the referral center for rural Nevada: the first stop. We could handle most of the cases, but often very complicated cases would have to be sent elsewhere. I remember a child with a brain tumor coming in from Winnemucca, and my friend and colleague, Dr. Charles Filippini, rode in the ambulance with the patient.

I did some assist work in operating rooms in our hospitals from time to time. One time—I don't know why, maybe they couldn't get anyone else—I was asked to assist Dr. John Ervin, a very nice man and fine surgeon. I was simply there to hold a retractor, but I don't know whether I was coming down with the flu or hadn't had anything to eat, but I said, "John, I've got to leave!" I thought I was going to pass out and I didn't know what the problem was. I had seen lots of blood over the years by assisting with C-sections, doing circumcisions, helping evacuate subdural hematomas, and drawing blood from subclavian veins, but on this case I almost lost it.

I used to go out with several pediatricians to rural areas and do consults. I remember one time driving to Yerington and visiting Dr. Mary Fulstone in her office. We would also go to doctors' offices in Fallon and other areas, and it was always a good break from my busy practice.

State-of-the-Art in Reno

Technology in Reno was state of the art when I came, and, now that I am retiring, I consider it an excellent medical community. Physicians and facilities could handle any medical contingencies that arise. One of the impressive advances was pulmonary equipment that could be set up in the home. It was called the pulmoaid machine and was very effective in treating kids with croup and asthma at home, keeping them out of emergency rooms and off the floors. I can remember long hours sitting in the ER at Washoe with the old BIRD machine, holding the kids and giving them a solution of vodka saline. We also would put the children in croup tents overnight and all of them would have to be admitted. Not too long afterwards, the University of Utah introduced a racemic epinephrine solution that was far more effective in alleviating symptoms.

Today we can treat those kids with Decadron and use the pulmoaid equipment in our offices. There have been new drugs introduced that save lives every day. We used to have to admit children with gastrointestinal problems and start IVs on them, but now we have solutions like Pedialyte that can relieve diarrhea problems quickly. Some of the children with acute diarrhea coming in from Schurz Indian reservation years ago, for example, were at death's door with stool shooting out of them.

It seems the consensus on whether or not to circumcise baby boys changes every few years. We know that in some cultures it is not looked upon favorably. The literature indicates that there is less penile cancer among circumcised men, but even that has been somewhat discredited. Then the argument comes up that the spread of AIDS is reduced when the man is circumcised. I honestly can't keep track. Dr. Penny Pemberton made it a practice not to do circumcisions at all, and I just don't know what is best.

There was a movement a while back in which women wanted to deliver their babies in water, and I always thought that was a terrible idea. Many of those babies would have to be put in the intensive care unit following water birthing because they developed breathing problems. One obstetrician who was just leaving the area when I arrived persuaded his mothers-to-be to deliver in the dark for some reason. That, too, I thought, was squirrely!

There have been many technological advances in my pediatric specialty over the years and I will try to name a few: broad spectrum antibiotics, surgical techniques for heart conditions, orthopedic surgery technology, allergies and asthma management, immunizations, and important advances in preventing birth defects and childhood injuries. Imaging technology advances also have been great. Infant and toddler car seats have improved, and laws have been changed to require "buckling up," which has prevented childhood injuries and saved lives.

I think I practiced during the best years of medicine even though the last few years were not all they could have been because managed care came in and changed everything, and not always for the better. I withheld joining any of the HMO and PPO-type plans until just recently.

Doctors have been taking the brunt of criticism about increased costs of health care for a long time now, while managed care administrators have been getting rich. The costs of prescription drugs is a big problem that has reached such a point that maybe only big government will be able to solve it. It really hit home when I learned first hand that meds and supplies for managing Type 2 diabetes can run $200 to $300 each month. That problem is being looked at in Washington right now, but the possible solutions suggested so far don't look like they will be helpful.

I've seen all these medical and technological improvements evolve over the years and have used them in my practice—and it was a wonderful practice. I am working part-time now and will begin to think about retiring when my medical malpractice insurance tail coverage begins sometime around the end of June this year.

Notes

[1] Jordon Crouch was a vice president of First National Bank, a leading banker in Nevada, and a prominent citizen in Reno.

[2] Donald W. Reynolds owned newspapers in Arkansas and was a financial contributor to the University of Nevada, Reno.

[3] Wesley W. Hall, M.D. was born in Mississippi in 1906. He was licensed from Reno in 1946 and practiced surgery until his retirement.

[4] William S. Keezer, M.D. was born in Indiana in 1919. He was licensed from Carson City in 1954 and practiced internal medicine and geriatrics.

[5] Roland W. Stahr, M.D. was born in Nebraska in 1901. He was licensed in Washoe County in 1939 and practiced pediatrics in Reno.

[6] John E. Palmer, M.D. was born in Winnemucca, Nevada, in 1915. He was licensed from Reno in 1945 and practiced pediatrics in Reno. William E. Pasutti, M.D. was born in Nevada in 1918. He was licensed from Reno in 1947 and practiced pediatrics in Reno. John G. Scott, Jr., M.D. was born in Pennsylvania in 1916. He was licensed in Reno in 1947 and practiced pediatrics in Reno. Emanuel Berger, M.D. was born in Czechoslovakia in 1903. He was licensed in Washoe County in 1949 and practiced pediatrics in Reno. William A. O'Brien III, M.D. was licensed in Nevada in 1947 and practiced anesthesiology.

13: Dr. John Iliescu, Plastic Surgery

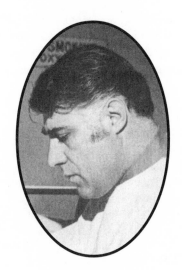

Dr. John Iliescu

Early Family

My mother and dad came from Romania, and I am a first generation American. My mother, Mary Russo, had eight siblings; her father was a town constable. She studied languages and her education was the equivalent of a college degree, which was a most remarkable feat during those times. My father only finished the fourth grade.

When my father was young, he was caught drinking wine, a product of the family vineyard. I was told he was punished so severely for it that he ran away to Egypt with a group of carpenters and worked there five or six years. He became a craftsman at cabinet making and returned later to Romania, where he met my mother. Uncle Ion Iliescu (my father's brother) served as president of Romania.

Realizing that America was a wonderful place of freedom, my parents decided this was the place to raise a family. My father had lived in the United States for a short time earlier before returning to Romania and marrying my mother. After immigrating to the United States via Ellis Island, they spent some time in New York City and then moved to Oak Park, Illinois, where I was born on August 26, 1926.

We were very close as a family as we had no other relatives in America. My mother was always the teacher, and my father, while stern, even a tyrant in many respects, always found time to spend with me and my siblings playing ball, ice skating, playing math games, and telling stories. My brother, George, died recently and was a remarkable man.

He was an accountant and a University of Illinois graduate, very soft-spoken and precise in his manner. My favorite sister, Helen, preceded George in death, dying here in Reno of respiratory failure, and I always thought of her as a true angel. My two other sisters, Florence and Eleanor, live in Reno.

Education

In school, I was content to sit on the back row and talk sports and such with my buddies, but my teacher seemed to realize I had potential and took an interest in me. She made me concentrate on math and encouraged me to play the violin. Mrs. Elliott would tolerate no nonsense and was quite firm, and in later years I realized she was just what I needed. I sent her roses when I finished dental school in appreciation for all she had done for me from the fifth to the eighth grades.

Times were very hard during the Great Depression. People had very little money and lots of people, including my father, who occasionally worked for the Work Progress Administration, were mostly unemployed. At Christmas time we always got baskets of food from the church. One time I remember an usher at church, spying the holes in my shoes, bought me a new pair.

I tried to earn extra money for the family by working for the milkman. I would get up a couple of hours before school and work from six until eight. And boy, those were some cold Chicago mornings. I had several other jobs up until I was fifteen or sixteen. I had a knack of getting along with people in every job. One of the jobs was delivering goods on my bicycle for Mr. Segal who owned five or six liquor stores and grocery stores in the area. All the money made in those jobs was given to my mother, who worked very hard taking in washing and ironing.

I went to Tilden Technical High School. It was the only such school in Chicago and students had to have fairly good grades to get admitted. Few students thought of going to college; in fact, technical high school was almost the equivalent of college. My mother wanted me to go. We didn't have money for that, but my dad was insistent I should learn a trade. I realized in later years that my lack of attention in school got me labeled as an average student, and this was probably one of the reasons I dropped out. The principle reason, however, came about as a result of my father breaking both his legs at the Work Progress Administration, and, without benefits, there was no other choice. I had to go to work.[1]

I got a job as an assistant lineman. As I was not afraid of heights, I was called "The Monkey" and got the job of scaling some pretty tall signs and such. I worked for about five or six months until my dad got well and then I joined the navy.

U.S. Navy

Since I was only seventeen years old, my parents had to sign for me. They thought that the war [World War II] would end before any of us volunteers would be shipped out, but it didn't end for two and a half years. After my first tour at Great Lakes Naval Station, I took some exams and became a radio technician. Later I went to the University of Chicago and learned how to become a frogman, and, as always, I managed to have fun in each assignment. On completion of my tour of duty, I had the chance to get an education. If there was anything I learned while in the navy, it was that getting an education was the only way. Fortunately the government did a wonderful thing in setting up the GI Bill. In Chicago they took a number of high schools with outstanding teachers and set up classrooms only for returning vets. Veterans could complete their high school education at their own speed and when they were finished, they could go down to the board of education and take a high school equivalency exam.

College and Dental School

In less than a year I was able to complete my high school education. I took two years of Latin and all the algebra and math courses required to go to college. On completion, I was asked from which high school I wanted my diploma and for sentimental reasons replied, "Well, let me go back to Tilden Tech. I'll take it from there."

I enrolled at the University of Illinois, where the tuition was quite reasonable, and began my first year in the engineering department on the Champagne campus. My second year was at the Cook County campus. I liked mathematics and physics even though I had so little of each in high school. My grades were quite good in those subjects. I finished a year at the University of Illinois in engineering and took a summer job in construction, got married, and about four or five months later found out my wife was pregnant with our first child, my daughter.

Within a short period of time though, I got an invitation to come to the University of Chicago for an interview. The dean had a reputation as being a very progressive educator. The entrance exam was divided into four parts. I did so very well on that exam, particularly the biology part, that I was encouraged to consider medicine, and since I had an interest in becoming a physician, this was most encouraging. My next year at the University of Chicago was in premed.

Requirements at that time were such that students had to have three years of undergraduate education before they could even apply for medical school. An "A" grade average, plus great recommendations, was the norm for entry. Even then, rumor had it that only one hundred out of a thousand applications were accepted.

We were having marital problems and my wife was convinced that if I went into medicine, she and my little daughter would never see me again. After we spent some time in marital counseling sessions, we agreed that dentistry was the field for me, and I applied and was accepted at the Illinois Dental School with the idea of specializing in orthodontics.

There were some very bright lights in the orthodontic program at Illinois, and I remember one of them, Dr. Bernie Sarnat, a dentist and medical doctor, was doing research on cleft palates, which fascinated me. I was accepted into his program and it didn't take long for me to decide that what I really wanted to do was plastic surgery. I got caught in the web.

Medical School

This presented yet another conflict in my life. I now wanted to go to medical school so I applied to half a dozen schools. I applied to Harvard, a very prestigious school that had recently developed a program in which they were awarding double degrees. Under their program, instead of taking four years to get through dental school and another four for med school, I could combine both and in seven years get both degrees. I got accepted and I was so excited I couldn't talk. I ran about a mile to tell a friend of mine. Only after reading the fine print and learning that Harvard prohibits medical students from working, I realized I would not be going there. It was quite an honor, however, to have been accepted in Harvard's medical-dental program. Soon afterwards I was accepted in the George Washington medical school program located in the District of Columbia and went to work for Illinois Senator Paul Douglas.

I was assigned to the police force in the rotunda of the senate office building. Hours were from five in the afternoon until eleven at night and this provided me with lots of time for study. This seemed to work well. There were also opportunities to earn extra money staffing social functions and guarding dignitaries. One such dignitary was the Queen of England on one of her visits to the area.

There was a growing problem, however. I wasn't seeing my family, and I missed my children; I had two when I entered medical school and one more by the time of my junior year. This absentee father business led to our divorce in 1962.

Internship and Residency

After medical school, I chose the University of Texas for my internship, and went to the Mayo Clinic for two years of the required three-year general surgery residency. I really enjoyed my work at the Mayo Clinic. It was quite academically oriented, and, at that time academia looked like a great career. I liked it there a lot. While quite strict, there was no high-pressure of any sort, and the mere mention of the Mayo Clinic in my resume opened lots of doors. I completed the third and final year of the general surgery residency at the University of California San Francisco before entering the plastic surgery training at Texas.

In my second year, I developed hepatitis as a result of a hypodermic needle stick and lost thirty pounds. I was quite sick for an awfully long time it seemed, and this convinced me that my considering academic medicine as a career was probably not going to work for me. I opted to study head and neck cancer, and I was trained at the M. D. Anderson Center in Texas.

While at the Mayo Clinic, I had a next-door neighbor named John Storm who hailed from Reno. Storm was a Daniel Boone type when it came to hunting and fishing, and we had done a lot of that during my stay at the clinic. I visited him occasionally over the years when he returned to Reno and fell in love with the place.

Plastic Surgery in Reno

The Move to Reno

I decided to come to Reno, stay with John Strom, look the place over, and come to some sort of decision on a place to start my practice. I had thought of going to either Reno or San Diego as both places had only one plastic surgeon. That was awfully hard for me to believe. When I came to Reno, I visited with Dr. Bill Champion and he said, "Well, there isn't really any room for another plastic surgeon. I'm only busy about sixty percent of the time." He told me the kinds of cases he was doing and those he wouldn't do. It was interesting; I was qualified and enjoyed doing all the procedures he preferred not to do. This was a wonderful challenge for me.

Dr. Jack Becker, a long-time orthopedic surgeon in Reno, had recently built a new medical office building at 1000 Ryland Street, and I think he had been having problems leasing space.[2] Some surgeons at WMC suggested I contact him. The building was basically empty with the exception of Dr. Becker on the fourth floor and a pharmacy and lab on the ground floor. I think he was shocked that day when I came to his office and asked him if I might sublet space. We negotiated, no, haggled over, the rental contract, finally settling for $150 per month.

Nevada License

The most immediate thing I had to do was to apply for a Nevada license through the Nevada Board of Medical Examiners. Dr. Kenneth Maclean was perennial chairman of the board and at the interview, he asked me lots of questions, strange questions like, was I going to charge outrageous prices for my services and whether or not I was a homosexual, but nothing about my training or medicine in general.

I told him that money was not my thing. I had come out of a university setting and didn't know much about making money, and that I would charge whatever the going rate was for my services. Furthermore, I would devote as much time as possible to indigent care. While there were other board members in the room, Ken did all the talking. He was a very dominant person, but the interview was carried out in a light manner, not too serious. Ken had a nice way about him: firm, but he never made me feel uncomfortable.

It didn't take me long to set up my practice, and I became busy right away. I didn't know anybody in town. The most cordial physicians to me were John Sande and Frank Russell.[3] John took me to lunch at the Nugget Oyster Bar within a few days of my opening practice. John was such a nice guy. He had dental and medical degrees and was doing quite a bit of plastic work. One would think that he would be the one person, as a competitor, who wouldn't be very friendly. Dr. Warren McClellan, a well-trained general surgeon in town, made me feel welcome and comfortable also. I remember one day he called me into the emergency room at Washoe County Hospital to assist him with a patient with a very severe facial laceration. The procedure, to my amazement, was done under a local anesthetic and it really should have been done in an operating room under general anesthesia. That was the way I was taught.

Medical Community in Reno

Other doctors I remember, who helped and encouraged me when I first started out, were Tom Kavanaugh, Don Mousel, V. A. Salvadorini, and Fred Stohl. Fred and I used to fly out to the "cow counties" in his private plane to do procedures, and more than once those flights were scary times for me.

At that time, St. Mary's Hospital was the facility in the area for elective plastic surgery. Dr. William Champion did not work at Washoe because they lacked the equipment he wanted. Even at Saints, Bill brought in his own surgical instruments. At Washoe I used surgical instruments borrowed from the eye or orthopedic sections. It was only later that plastic surgery equipment and instruments were bought by the hospital.

There were two groups of anesthesiologists in town and a healthy competition had developed over the years between the two. If one worked exclusively with one group, members of the other group were reluctant to come out in the middle of the night to work with them. That was just the way it was. I developed an excellent relationship with anesthesiologist Massoud Dorostkar, who, like me, was just starting out building his practice. He volunteered to provide anesthesia for my patients virtually twenty-four hours a day and I really appreciated that. I used him almost exclusively for the next twenty years. He knew all my quirks and mannerisms, like my policy of always being in the room when my patients were put to sleep.

Building a medical practice in Reno was like walking on eggs; it was really tough. I can remember working with certain doctors in town who had big egos in certain respects. They did not take kindly to suggestions at all. I let a doctor assist me in surgery one time and saw he was pulling too hard on the suturing tissue. I asked him not to do it that way and he got offended. After that, I developed my own surgical team.

I brought new technology into town with me and this placed some of the doctors who continued to do plastic and reconstructive work at a disadvantage. They were put in a position of continuing to do procedures out of their field of expertise when there was a new, highly trained specialist available in the area.

Reno physicians were acutely aware of the monetary side of medical practice and guarded it furiously at times. The medical school coming to town was a good example. Reno doctors were not all that certain that starting a medical school was such a good idea and some of them did put up a protest, but mostly behind the scenes.

Carroll Ogren, administrator of WMC, was helpful in getting all the equipment and instruments I needed and was very supportive of my building my surgical team there. Since Dr. Champion preferred to do all his work at St. Mary's hospital, I dedicated myself to building the plastic surgery section at WMC. In hospital management everything comes down to money. As I steadily built my practice at Washoe, I could get almost anything I needed. I would give Carroll a list periodically, and I got those items almost immediately. Ogren was a really smart and nice man, and an excellent administrator.

He always appreciated that my procedures were done on time. A lot of surgeons in those days would ask for four hours but take only two hours, while others would ask for two and take four hours. That would upset the operating room scheduling and the whole surgical floor.

Over the years, my colleagues in private practice would ask about my office staff wondering if I had experienced theft of any kind. I was often asked, "Well John, how do you know your help is not stealing from you?" I had heard about office theft often enough, but I never gave it a second thought in my own office. If that sort of thing did occur, I didn't want to know about it—it's too late now anyway.

Over the years I had wonderful office staff and one of the first ladies I employed, Joann Freshour, was with me for five years and did an enormous amount of quality work for me. In fact, when she left and married a dentist up in Winnemucca, I had to hire three women to replace her. She was very honest and did everything.

One day I had to fire all three of those women I had just hired because they couldn't get the work done. I began advertising for a replacement and the first lady I interviewed was Dr. Jack Flanary's sister-in-law, Jo Lynn Flanary. I went on to interview about fifty other applicants, but Jo Lynn kept popping into my mind. I was concerned about hiring someone so closely associated with the physician community because Reno was a small town and office gossip abounded. After all the interviews were completed, I contacted Jo Lynn and offered her the job. Although she had taken another position in a local dentist's office, she accepted my offer and gave her two weeks notice. She was with me for twenty-five years.

Burn Center at WMC

When I came to this community and started practicing in February 1970, all burns were sent out of the area, over the mountain so to speak, and they had to be transported by ground ambulance. When I arrived, I saw most of the massive burn trauma in the emergency room. I had trained in a very large burn center, probably the largest in America at that time, and my experiences were extensive. I remember being called an SOB more than once. SOB stands for Supervisor of Burns, which means having total responsibility of all burn management in the facility. Of course, I had a staff of people working day and night because this is one of the most intense specialties in medicine.

Reno hospitals were not treating burns, as no one was trained, and every burn patient was shipped out. Carroll Ogren and I felt we had the potential to effectively treat burns, and, since I had three years intensive burn treatment experience, we established a team of wonderful nurses and community volunteers and set up the first burn unit in northern Nevada.

I take none of the credit for that; I was just a member of a dynamic team. Through it all, it was a very emotional choking experience to think about the devotion everyone gave to patients and to this program. There were times when we had children burned so badly we used every vein we could find to start intravenous fluid lines to supplement their fluid intake. We'd soon run out of them and we'd have to use their scalp and their jugular veins. I mean, one would have to be really creative to try to find ways to care for them. We were not always successful either.

General surgeons, as a rule, did not want to take care of burns. In fact, plastic surgeons, those who were not trained as I was, didn't really like it all that much. It is a twenty-four hour, seven-day a week job. In my case I was used to it. I came out of that kind of training program, plus, I was spending so many hours at the hospital with emergency trauma and was up all night operating anyway. It was not hard for me to go in frequently to look in on my burn patients and see how they were doing.

Treating burns is a highly complicated business. The technology at that time was surprisingly state of the art with what it is today. Grafts using skin from the patient, the patient's twin, a cadaver, or donor pigs, and a technique called mesh grafting, were as common then as now. Scarring was a huge problem in treating burn patients then and it still is now.

Over the years treating burn patients has evolved to a point where we have been able to grow skin in the laboratory. That skin effectively covers large areas on a badly burned patient and this has been a big step forward in treatment. Unfortunately, lab produced tissue is not as good as normal skin and has its complications, but, in most instances it is life saving and works quite well. Tissue grafts have been used in Reno probably for the past ten years, and the basic technique in treating burns haven't changed all that much. We still have to get the patient through the acute stage, watch the fluid intake and output, and cover the area.

Within eight or nine years after the burn center was established at WMC, a very large center was set up at the University of California in San Francisco and Care Flight (helicopter) services were made available in northern Nevada. A liability would be imposed on us if we treated patients for severe burns and they died when there was a comprehensive burn center only a short flight away. With that in mind, we dismantled the unit and began shipping critical burn patients to San Francisco. One important observation has to be made: treating burns at Washoe was never a moneymaker; only the large burn centers pay their own way.

Move to St. Mary's Hospital

As time went on, I eventually took more and more of my practice to St. Mary's; in fact, I spent almost all my time there the last fifteen years of my career. Excellent outpatient surgery facilities developed at Saints, which made it easy for many of my patients. They could have surgery, a face-lift for example, and go home the same day. Certainly, with breast augmentation, they would go home the same afternoon. Much of my cosmetic work was done on an "in and out basis."

Advances in Plastic Surgery

A question comes up regarding doing some of the major cosmetic procedures in the physicians' offices because many plastic surgeons began doing just that many years ago. I don't think I did one percent of my surgeries in my office. It was all done at the hospital, as I always felt it was safer for the patient. If an emergency came up, what could be better than to have an entire hospital staff and facilities standing by? Patients, too, were becoming aware that a doctor who did all his surgeries in his office just might not have hospital privileges with all the checks, balances, and credentialing required.

There have been impressive advances in technology, instrumentation, and pharmaceuticals used by plastic surgeons in recent years. The use of lasers was a big step forward and fiberoptics have come in to play. Now, face-lifts, forehead surgeries, and surgery of the nasolabial area can be done through smaller incisions with a fiberoptic scope, just like general surgeons use for removal of gallbladders. But, those are just tools of the trade. The basic principles haven't really changed that much. We are still doing, by way of those extra tools, basically the same thing we did through a larger incision to achieve the same type of results.

Antibiotics have really changed things for general surgeons and have certainly provided benefits for plastic surgery. Modern antibiotics created situations so that closure of a severe wound could be delayed for several days. We could clean up debris, compress the area, and wait until the swelling was reduced. Then, we could clearly see all the tissue before closing. One would get a nicer job. Facial fractures could be repaired the same way—using antibiotics effectively.

My career as a plastic and reconstructive surgeon in Reno was a most fulfilling and satisfying one, and I can hardly believe I have retired. I would still consider doing academic medicine of some sort if the opportunity arose, but if it doesn't, that's okay too. My time in Reno has been just wonderful, and I have enjoyed my many friends, colleagues, and the support of the community all along the way.

Notes

[1] WPA designates Roosevelt's New Deal's Works Progress Administration (WPA) to provide work for those on dole.

[2] Dr. John C. Becker was born in Reno, Nevada, in 1916 and licensed in Nevada in 1948

[3] Dr. Frank Russell was born in California in 1915 and licensed in Nevada in 1946.

14: Dr. John Chappel, Psychiatry

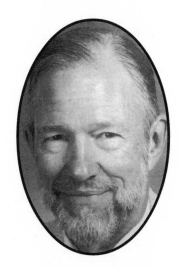

Dr. John Chappel

Born in Canada

I was born November 5, 1931, in Grand Prairie, Alberta, Canada right in the heart of the Great Depression. As a western Canadian, I was quite comfortable relocating to Reno later in my career. There had been two physicians who were anesthesiologists, in my mother's family and both served in World War II. Looking back, I don't think they were role models for me in my decision to go into medicine, as my chief encouragement came from my immediate family. Dad was a Methodist minister in the United Church of Canada and there was plenty of encouragement from him, from the very beginning, for me to get as much professional education as possible.

My dad's work in the ministry meant we moved quite a bit. Before he went into the military, we had moved to three different provinces and when he returned, we moved to Toronto where he worked for the Canadian Council of Christian Education. His work took him to New York where he served as General Secretary of the World Council of Christian Education, but I was incensed that the family would be abandoning Canada so I stayed and started classes at the Ontario Veterinarian College. In my second year, one of my classmates attempted suicide and none of us knew what to do, but we thought somebody ought to stay with him. I studied with him and it turned out that he knew more than I did about the basic sciences that we were studying. However, he would go into the examinations and I would come out near the top of the class and he would be at the bottom. That baffled me so much that I went to the University of Alberta, my parents' alma mater, and began a course of study in clinical psychology.

An Interest in Psychology

After doing a graduate year in clinical psychology and working in a child-guidance clinic, I observed that psychiatrists on the staff had most of the influence even though they seemed to know less about personalities than those studying psychology. As I looked at my classmates studying for their doctorate degrees in psychology and taking such a long time to complete their dissertations, I felt that becoming a medical doctor might well be easier so I started medical school in 1956. I enrolled in the University of Alberta Medical School with interest in psychiatry; I quickly got turned off by the Department of Psychiatry and switched my studies to general practice.

Medical Practice and Psychiatry

I spent a year in general practice in rural Alberta and then joined CARE/MEDICO and worked in Malaysia from 1962 to 1964. It was from these experiences that I decided that community psychiatry interested me most. I obtained a U.S. Public Health Service fellowship and enrolled in the Harvard School of Public Health. Later, I entered residency training in psychiatry at the University of Chicago under the tutelage of Dr. Knight Aldridge, chairman of the department.

An Interest in Addiction Treatment

After completing that program in 1968, I was invited to be medical director of the heroin detoxification ward at the University of Chicago and was there six years. We had twelve thousand heroin addicts in treatment at one time and it was one of the biggest programs in the country. It was a huge program in a very complex area of medicine.

It was a confusing time in drug addiction treatment. As many as eighty percent of the soldiers and sailors coming home from Vietnam had drug addiction problems and programs were set up to provide treatment before they reached home. At the same time, a lot of attention was being paid to prescribing practices of physicians and the treatment programs. We discovered, to our chagrin, that addicts would be treated, get "cleaned up," and be directed to find a primary care physician for their continued medical care. As soon as the doctors discovered they were heroin addicts, our patients were either treated badly or were refused treatment altogether. Interestingly, there was no coherent training in addiction medicine in any medical schools in the country at that time. This was probably a result of the Harrison Act, passed by congress in

1914, and the Prohibition Amendment passed in 1919. These attempts to rid the country of alcohol and other drugs surgically excised training in alcohol or drug addiction from medical school curricula. At that time, there seemed to be a consensus that drug addicts were bad people, and, if physicians prescribed for them, they, too, were bad people. Some doctors used opiates in their treatment of drug addicts and a number were arrested and incarcerated in the early 1920s for doing that. This sent a chill throughout the medical profession for a long time.

Move to the Faculty of the University of Chicago

Dr. Jerry Jaffe recruited me to the faculty of the University of Chicago. President Richard Nixon later appointed him to head up the war on drugs in 1971, and he became the first drug czar. He was a very forward-thinking individual who developed his ideas when he worked at prison hospitals in Lexington, Kentucky, and Ft. Worth, Texas. When Jaffe went to Washington as drug czar, he established the first big treatment program for Vietnam veterans, which started before they arrived home. Jaffe believed that drug addicts needed to have multi-modality treatment and we established a variety of treatment modalities for this purpose. He suggested that they needed to be treated in the communities where they lived.

Jaffe set up the detoxification units with mandatory urine drug screening of all servicemen who were going to be sent home and got them detoxed and treated before they came back. It turned out to work very well because the ones who had never used drugs before didn't return to using drugs once they were home. For some reason there was an enormous fear of what drug-addicted soldiers would do when they came home. I was lucky getting in at the very beginning of this innovative addiction treatment concept. Then along came the National Institute on Alcoholism and Alcohol Abuse (NIAAA), the National Institute on Drug Abuse, (NIDA), and the Controlled Substances Act, which placed prescription drugs in different classes depending on their propensity for addiction. Schedule I drugs were deemed to be the most addictive and the most dangerous. It included marijuana, heroin, and LSD. Physicians were not allowed to prescribe them. Schedule II were prescription drugs for narcotics and had to be hand-written, were non- refillable, and required triplicate forms. Schedules III, IV, and V drugs had addictive potential but to a lesser degree.

Before these changes in medical education began to take effect, medical schools had produced several generations, certainly several decades, of physicians ignorant about addictive disorders. One of the programs Jaffe set up was a career teacher program in alcohol and drugs, which was designed to identify a senior faculty member in each medical school who would introduce addition medicine in the curriculum. This was called the Career Teacher Program in Alcohol and Drug Abuse, and it interested me a great deal. It became clear at the University of Chicago, however, that I could have stayed on in this capacity indefinitely but I never would have gotten tenure. So I started looking for places to go and my hope was that I would be able to go back to Canada but that just didn't happen. I looked at different schools and my wife and I chose five places to visit—one being Reno.

Psychiatry in Reno

The Move to the University of Nevada School of Medicine

One of the bright lights in psychiatry, Paul Miller, M.D., had become chair of the Division of Behavioral Sciences at the newly created two-year medical school at the University of Nevada. Paul had been on the faculty at Northwestern and was recruited by University of California, Davis medical school. He was very interested in the psychiatric aspects of creativity and developed a case history using the life of Vincent van Gogh, a prime example of a very creative but disturbed individual. Paul thought this might be a very good training case to present to medical students and to physicians to show the way in which mental illness affects people. Van Gogh was severely depressed and eventually killed himself, probably due to drug related changes in his brain caused by drinking alcohol and turpentine. Paul showed, through pictures and paintings, how isolated this artist was; how he couldn't get along with anybody, and through his paintings and with the song, "*Starry, Starry Night*," recorded by singer Don McLean, offered a program for medical students on mental illness that was fascinating. Van Gogh was analyzed in this innovative fashion over his entire lifespan.

Paul thought of this as an introduction to psychopathology for the medical students. I saw it as a great introduction not only for that, but to addiction medicine as well.

I came to Reno and talked with Paul and Dean George Smith at the school and then went to Stanford for a recruiting visit. The Chairman of the Psychiatry Department there asked who the competition was. When I said, "the University of Nevada," he commented, "Nevada! Do they have a medical school? My fantasy is that there will be a number of desks out amongst the sagebrush in the desert."

If I had gone to Stanford, it would have been a repeat of what I had experienced at the University of Chicago and that was minimal influence on the curriculum. All we were allowed to do was teach elective courses. There were a hundred medical students in the class at the University of Chicago at the time and we would get, at best, two to five students in each class who showed any interest at all in addiction medicine.

After my visit to Stanford, my wife, Valerie, and I visited three places in Canada. Alberta wanted me to be medical director of their provincial programs, but the University of Alberta had no interest in addiction medicine. My wife and I considered the medical schools in Ottawa and Toronto too stuffy. Dean George Smith and Paul Miller offered a required week in the second year of medical school. Although it was less money, it was the best teaching opportunity and I accepted a position at the two-year University of Nevada School of Medical Sciences in 1974.

Teaching in Reno
Nevada used an organ block system in the two-year program and there were six weeks for the central nervous system coordinated by physiologist Matt Bach. I was offered a full week in that block for addiction medicine.

In the beginning there was no time for building any sort of private practice. Paul Miller was interested in developing a consultation-type practice and we did some of that at the VA, at the Nevada Mental Health Institute, and for the Washoe Association for Retarded Citizens (WARC). It was quite an experience because Paul was a driving, energetic individual. He became incensed by clinical psychologists at the school not working as hard as he did. He attempted to have one of them fired. This was unacceptable and Dean Smith relieved him as chairman of the department, and moved him into the Dean's office for a year. Paul then moved to the Auburn, California, for a while; then he moved to the Los Angeles area where he lives and works today, teaching part-time at UCLA. This was an example of one of those painful lessons we all learn: you can't bring into any organization the attitude of being the sole decision maker. No matter how legitimate you may think your decisions are, if they are not supported by the organization, you will be the one to go.

There were several outstanding mental health professionals practicing at the school when I came: DeWitt "Bud" Baldwin, M.D., had been in the area for some time and became the first chairman of the department at the fledgling School of Medical Sciences; Dan Oppleman, Ed.E., and Dan Tone helped us a lot from the Division of Educational Support and Communication (DESC); John Altrocchi, Ph.D., and Bill Hudspeth, Ph.D., were also in the department, and Jerry May, Ph.D., preceded me by a month or two. Hudspeth was a clinical psychologist who did electroencephalographic studies of glucose metabolism and insulin. I think Bill left before we became a four-year school.

Psychiatry at WMC

Another psychiatrist practicing in the area was Dr. Dick Gilmore. He was a crusty, opinionated older psychiatrist who was chief of staff in psychiatry at Washoe Medical Center where Miller and I had privileges. One of the first things I did when I came to town was to gain staff privileges at Washoe, and I have been on the staff ever since. We worked at Station 18, the psychiatric ward at the hospital, and Gilmore called all the shots. One of his policies was quite unusual: he wouldn't allow any clergy on the psychiatric ward. He thought they disrupted psychiatric treatment, so priests, rabbis, ministers, and pastors were not allowed to come in to see members of their congregation who had been admitted there. Even more interesting than his position prohibiting clergy from working on the ward was the fact that clergy members did not object. There was passivity among them. Clergy are used to visiting hospitalized patients on the medicine and surgery floors. Perhaps they considered physical trauma not to involve a patient's belief system, their thinking and emotions as frequently happens when mental illness is involved.

I think Gilmore reflected in an almost extreme way what had happened in medical education in the nineteenth century. Religion had been taken out of medical education and practice. It was viewed as being something that ought not to interfere with good medical care. If you saw a patient who had a different religious persuasion than your own, you didn't attack that, you respected it and you didn't allow it to interfere with your medical care. Freud, himself, would challenge religion and thought a lot of it was delusional, so there was an almost agnostic or atheistic view of religion by psychiatry.

Over the years there has been a continuing interest by psychiatrists in religion. At its annual meeting, the American Psychiatric Association usually has one or more programs on this subject.

Pain Control

Another of my interests is helping patients with chronic pain, who have been "fired" by pain doctors in town. When that occurs, it is mostly due to behavioral problems. The pain doctors put their patients on strict regimens. If those patients disregard those strict regimens and go to emergency rooms for pain relief or seek out other physicians for medications, they will be "fired." Pain doctors have long waiting lists of patients wanting to enter their programs. Some of those patients end up in my department. Fortunately we have a certified substance abuse counselor who is interested in chronic pain as well as in the different forms of addiction.

Reno's Psychiatrists

Dr. Les Gould was a psychiatrist in town when I arrived. He traveled to Elko every month to see patients at the Mental Health Center. Les eventually married the nurse who was the supervisor of Station 18 at Washoe Med. The Nevada Division of Mental Health and Mental Retardation, as it used to be called, had just established centers in the larger towns. These included Elko, Winnemucca, Fallon, Yerington, and Hawthorne. When Les developed cancer and was not able to go to Elko, the division recruited me to take his place. I flew out once a month in one of those little cigar box planes that was later replaced by larger craft operated by Hughes Air West. Passengers called it "Scare West."

Don Molde, M.D., was another psychiatrist who came into town about the same time I did. He was very much a presence in the psychiatry community. I think he and Les Gould were in practice together for a while.

Another physician, Dr. Gene Montgomery, practiced in Reno during the mid 1970s and was responsible for one of the most dramatic and shocking events in the community. He appeared calm and competent, but was a very disturbed man who later killed his wife and himself with a shotgun. It turned out that he was receiving psychiatric treatment away from the Reno community and as so often happens, distant treatment does not work well. Physicians with mental problems do much better by getting treatment in the same community in which they practice. He, like many psychiatrists, tended to be socially and politically isolated; this may have to do with the kind of personalities that are attracted into psychiatry.

Psychiatric Evaluations on Inmates

I also got involved with the courts and with doing evaluations for inmates and mental patients. I once evaluated the man who, oddly enough, was responsible for the development of the Lake's Crossing program. He was from a well-known family in northern Nevada, had been treated at the Nevada Mental Health Institute, and had paranoid schizophrenia. He did well when he was on his medications, but when he was sent home, he apparently stopped taking his medications and developed a delusion that his parents were going to harm him in some way. He got a knife and killed them both. He was a high profile individual and the Nevada Mental Health Institute did not have enough security to treat him safely, so he was sent over to California to the prison hospital at Vacaville. The money they charged the State of Nevada was such that the legislature decided to build Lake's Crossing, as a secure hospital treatment program.

I worked there doing evaluations for close to ten years. There was scant time to have a private practice, but I was doing quite a lot of clinical work at the Veterans Administration Hospital. Dr. Paul Miller and the department wanted to make the VAH a site for medical student training, and the administration at the hospital was supportive.

The Reno Veterans Administration Hospital

The VA had one clinical psychologist, Dick Blurton, who was providing mental healthcare at the hospital when Paul first came to town. We worked hard with Dick to develop a program and recruited Ed Lynn, M.D., as the first psychiatrist to head up the mental health service there. Ed was very much involved in medical education and followed Paul Miller as chairman of the department for a brief period. Today he is practicing in Carson City.

UNSOM and a Psychiatic Society

About this same time there was a groundswell to make the University of Nevada School of Medical Sciences into a full four-year institution. I think the intent from the very beginning had been to have a four-year school as soon as it was politically and financially possible. I can't say there was great concern exhibited by local psychiatrists for this to happen; in fact, there was little or no interest. There was local support, however, for development of a psychiatric association in Reno, which could promote interest in mental health and psychiatry as a discipline.

Some of the psychiatrists were upset by what was happening at the Nevada Mental Health Institute. There appeared to be a systematic plan to replace psychiatrists with clinical psychologists. Charles Dixon, who had a doctorate in clinical psychology, had been made director of the institute and had published an article suggesting that psychiatric patients just needed humane treatment. Maybe the state would do better by spending those psychiatric therapy funds to send those patients to Hawaii for vacation treatment. That was like waving a red flag in front of a bull. Don Molde took the lead in publicly objecting to such comments and thinking. He was very active in organized medicine and politics through his work as president of the Washoe County Medical Society and his legislative lobbying efforts. He worked on the county and state levels of organized medicine to reverse this trend and I think he made good progress. Realistically, he understood that there was an ample supply of psychologists who could be employed for about half the cost of psychiatrists, and this situation would be very difficult to reverse.

The political scene bears continuous watching and I have been supportive of the political efforts the AMA has made over the years and have always been a member. While I was at the University of Chicago, the chief of internal medicine called me in one day to explore the reason why I was only one of five physicians on the faculty who was also a member of the AMA. He was very supportive and he wanted me to encourage our students and residents to get involved with organized medicine as soon as they could. I did my part while there and here at UNSOM, but it has always been obvious that academic physicians tend to shun organized medicine.

Psychiatric Drugs

When I was a general practitioner, there were several drugs that came the scene and proved effective in treating various forms of mental illness. Thorazine was available, which I seldom used in my general practice, but which, from the literature, showed great promise in psychiatry. I think the first of the benzodiazepines and antidepressants had come out and I used to prescribe a lot of those, including imipramine, doxepin, chlordiazepoxide, and diazepam. These were mainstays in the armamentarium of GPs and psychiatrists in mental health treatment back then. There were several central nervous system depressants available and they were the precursors of Xanax, Ativan, and Klonipin. I prescribed a lot of these drugs and they worked quite well.

I was not involved in the mental health arena when I first entered practice as a GP, but Thorazine and the subsequent medications.resulted in dramatic change and improvement in mental treatment. Across the nation, we saw wards at most of the state hospitals being emptied out. This was the beginning of the use of a growing list of medications that made it possible for people to be hospitalized for relatively short periods of time even though they might have severe, chronic, disabling psychiatric disorders.

Electroconvulsive Therapy

Electroconvulsive therapy (ECT) was used in the 1960s, but it was going through some difficult political times. I remember later in the 1980s, our psychiatric community had a debate about this procedure and there was a doctor who had published a book called, *Toxic Psychiatry*, in which he attacked not only ECT and its use, but also all these medications as being toxic to the brain. He made his points, but by then the horse was already out of the barn as these drugs were in widespread use, and their effectiveness was making an enormous difference in psychiatric practice.

Lobotomies

In the earlier days of psychiatry, doctors did more frontal lobotomies. These were quite crude procedures. There were no stereotactic measurements and guidelines for surgery as there are today. Psychosurgery has never been very popular among mental health professionals, as it tends to be destructive and disruptive of the normal brain circuitry. Proper medications are more effective and much easier to deal with. Psychosurgery is still done in some areas of the country, but to my knowledge it has never been done in northern Nevada, or southern Nevada for that matter.

Psychiatrists are seldom called in to assist in any form of brain or other surgery, but I have been called in after surgery to assist with patients who were being detoxed when they come out of anesthesia and were going into delirium tremens.

Political Issues

Psychiatrists and psychologists generally get along very well except when it comes to political issues. Over the years relationships between the two groups have been tense in northern Nevada and this tension has spilled over on several levels. Dr. Jerry May, who later became associate dean of student affairs at the school, was the third clinical psychologist who came into the medical school department. He joined the faculty within a month after I came. We have been contemporaries and good friends every since.

The Section of Psychiatry and Behavioral Sciences has been very fortunate in having a series of high quality chairs who were both energetic and competent. After Drs. Bud Baldwin and Paul Miller, we recruited Ed Lynn. When he left, we did a national search as the school became a full-fledged, four-year medical school. Ira Pauly, M.D., came from the University of Oregon Medical School. Under his leadership we developed a fully-accredited residency in psychiatry. Many of the graduates of this program are now practicing psychiatrists in Nevada.

When Ira retired in 1994, we mounted another national search and Ole Thienhaus, M.D., from the University of Cincinatti became our chair. Under his leadership our department increased its activities in southern Nevada and a residency program has been approved for Las Vegas. To my knowledge, Ole is the first chair of any department in the medical school to successfully manage two separate programs: one in Reno and one Las Vegas.

I never was one of leaders, but I have been privileged to play a role in selecting our leadership. I chaired the search committee which selected Bob Daugherty, M.D., to be the dean of our newly-accredited, four-year medical school. I also served as acting chair of psychiatry three times after Drs. Paul Miller, Ed Lynn, and Ira Pauly. Fortunately, the department survived my administrative ineptitude.

Another political issue has been the relationship between psychiatrists and psychologists. While there have been few direct confrontations, there has been a great deal of concern by physicians about psychologists gaining admitting privileges at psychiatric hospitals or the ability to prescribe psychiatric medications. That battle is fought every biennium in the Nevada legislature and has been the major area of conflict. These disputes are not limited to mental health professionals, as legislative fights are legend among orthopedists/chiropractors, ophthalmologists/optometrists, and the desire of certain dental specialties to have hospital privileges to extract teeth and do oral surgery.

Psychiatrists and their colleagues in family practice and pediatrics have consistently been on the bottom rungs of the medical earnings ladder. It has been a battle to get third party payers to place more value on cognitive processes and intellectual services. All of us have benefited from changes in Medicare.

Mental Health Professionals

Our department has always been committed to having faculty from the major mental health professions, particularly clinical psychology. Both Jerry May, and John Altrocchi were advoca=tes of that policy. We also worked with Dr. Dick Blurton, chief of mental health services at the VAH. We effected policies to assure that the mental health service was staffed by both clinical psychologists and psychiatrists.

The VAH has developed as a major teaching facility for clinical psychology. A lot of the students and faculty of the psychology department at the University have done their internship at the VAH. We've had a very tenuous relationship with the UNR psychology faculty over the years. For a while, we were invited to give lectures there and we invited graduate students in psychology to audit classes of interest to them, but this has waxed and waned and has mostly waned over the last decade or two. I've been here almost three decades. We do have a joint research project on smoking cessation, and the UNR Department of Psychology has done the clinical work in our department, but it has not been a close relationship.

Retirement

When we moved to Reno, we got a house on McDonald Drive, and all three of my children completed schooling at public schools—they were all good schools. I only had one child, a daughter, who showed an interest in a medical education, but her MCAT scores were a bit low and she was advised to take some time to concentrate on improving those scores. She, however, became interested in a career in music and started singing for a living as she considered singing much more fun than medicine. Laura Chappel works with a group called "Whitewood" and has made an excellent name for herself in northern Nevada. All my children have settled in the Reno area and my wife and I continually enjoy our six grandchildren.

I think Reno is one of the best places in the world to live. Unfortunately more people are discovering that fact. But it is also apparent that we are not being swamped as Las Vegas has been. It was interesting to watch the effect of the MGM when it first was built, back in the early 1980s, as that was the time the infrastructure in Reno became initially stressed and couldn't keep up with the influx of people, but it's done pretty well since then.

I retired from full-time faculty when I turned sixty-five in 1997. I then went on a Letter of Appointment for teaching and practicing at the medical school. I am still doing the same teaching I was doing. Fortunately, the school has recruited a new, young psychiatrist, Mark Broadhead, who joined the staff and has an interest in addiction medicine. He is co-teaching with me at present and will be gradually taking over those teaching aspects there. I have a part-time practice in addiction medicine within the department and I do general psychiatry as well.

One of the things that has happened to me in this active "retirement" business is that I have been selected to be medical director of West Hills Hospital in Reno. So, here we go again. It seems I will have my hand in psychiatric medicine, in some capacity, for many more years to come.

I have had a wonderful practice in a fascinating specialty and have been particularly fortunate to have such a fine, state-of-the-art medical community. We have lived in a wonderful part of the country. The medical school has made a substantial contribution, not only to the medical profession, but also to the Reno community. My wife and I have made so many lifetime friends here and we have been blessed with happy and healthy children and grandchildren. What more could we ask for?

15: Dr. Frederick Boyden, Radiology

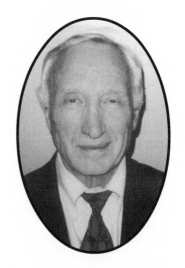

Dr. Frederick Boyden

Early Life and Education

I was born August 12, 1935, in Schuyler, Nebraska, and raised in Tecumseh, a small town in the southeastern part of the state. My father worked for the county as an agricultural agent and my mother was a high school math teacher. There weren't any medical people in my family and I had no interest throughout my high school days in going into medicine. My time at Hastings College, about a hundred miles west of Lincoln, was spent trying to live up to my basketball scholarship. It didn't take very long to realize I was never going to be a wage earner in that field.

In the middle of my sophomore year, my English teacher called me aside and asked me what I wanted to do with my life. I said, "Well, I will probably be a coach or whatever, I don't really have any direction." She said, "Well, the people who work with you in chemistry and physics think you would make a good physician and there is going to be a "Premed Day" in Omaha coming up and they thought you should go down and take a look." So I went down to the big city of Omaha and saw people I had known from Hastings who had gone into medicine and asked them how it was. They said it really wasn't that tough and that they would really like to see me come—they thought that it would be a good profession for me.

I went back to Hastings and was playing Ping-Pong with a good friend, Dick Cottingham. He noticed I was wavering on making a decision so, in front of a fairly large crowd in the student union, he said, "This is Fred Boyden from Tecumseh, Nebraska, and he doesn't have the guts to go to medical school." I went around the table after him and I said, "The hell I don't." I went and checked in with my advisor and was on my way to a career in medicine.

A Medical Career

I completed my premed courses at Hastings and entered medical school at Nebraska in 1956, graduating in 1960. Another Nebraska medical school classmate is Dr. Jack Talsma, who has had an excellent career in ophthalmology here in Reno.

I did my internship at Los Angeles County Hospital and got a well-rounded education in treating heart attacks, bleeding ulcers, and lots of trauma. LA County was called "The King of all Hospitals" for trauma. During that intern year, I met my wife, Jeanne, who had also been born in Nebraska and was now living in Long Beach; not too many months later we married. Jeanne and my parents were good friends and this union was almost like an arranged marriage.

U.S. Navy and Radiology

My military duty was served with the U.S. Navy in Taiwan from 1961-1963, where Jeanne and I had Eric and Jenny, our two oldest children. I had been a navy reservist back in Nebraska beginning in 1953 and served those two years in Taiwan as a lieutenant.

I still didn't know quite what I wanted to do for a career in medicine. When I returned to the states, I spent a year at Shasta County Hospital in Redding, California, and began looking around at several family practice possibilities. None of these seemed to fit very well.

I called a radiology resident friend of mine, Dr. Ken Moorhead, in Denver who said, "Fred, go into radiology, you are going to love it. We are getting into angiography and invasive procedures. Just take my word. You'll like it, and we just so happen to have a spot open." He pointed out that I had already gotten my military obligation out of the way and he could guarantee me that I'd get the position. I got the job and spent the next three years in radiology residency at the University of Colorado.

Radiology in Reno

The Move to Reno

Why did I select Reno? Well, my in-laws were in Long Beach and I was from Nebraska. I wanted to be close to them, but not too close; a one-hour flight was just right.

The thing that enticed me to settle here was that Washoe Medical Center was opening up a brand new building and radiology facility, and furthermore, I liked all the partners in the group. In addition, a new medical school was in the wings. When the medical school opened, I was one of the physicians who volunteered to teach. I was asked to give lectures in concert with medical school staff, and I have continued to do this from my current position at the VA.

I also enjoyed the area. I was very impressed with the administrator at Washoe, Carroll Ogren, who was a very fine hospital administrator. I knew it was going to be a top-of-the-line hospital. Carroll became one of my good friends, and he was on top of every situation. He would make morning rounds and eliminate potential problems by "nipping them in the bud." In addition, I had gotten to know Dr. Ernie Mack, chairman of the Washoe Board of Directors and he was always very helpful. Carroll and Dr. Mack had planned extra floors in the new building in anticipation of growth in the community. They knew of the need for more beds and there would have to be room for new services and the most advanced equipment.

Radiology Practice

The radiologists who impressed me back in 1967 when I interviewed in town were Drs. Lee Sandars, who was the senior radiologist, Don Hlubucek, and Bill Feltner. In those days, radiologists were trained in both radiation therapy and diagnosis. I, along with Dr. Bill Feltner, opened the first cobalt treatment unit in town in 1969. We did radiation therapy for about ten years, and then I passed into the shadows in therapy and continued to do only diagnostic radiology. When I came, Washoe had a "red goggle" radiology department. We all wore red goggles when we did fluoroscopy to accommodate our eyes for the darkness. The need for goggles gradually faded with the advent of new equipment.

I actually performed the first catheter angiogram in the state in 1967 and have been a "needler" and invasive radiologist for years, so this seems to fit. Since then, I probably have performed somewhere between four and five thousand angiograms and was the only show in town for a long time. We all shared that duty, but today people are specifically trained in subspecialties and invasive work. I was gradually limited, being the only member with no fellowship training in the invasive end of radiology.

Turf battles were notorious then, and continue to be. The original "coronary angiogram" was performed by Dr. Mel Judkins at Loma Linda University, and I had the opportunity to work with him for three or four weeks. I came back and felt quite comfortable doing that procedure, but lo and behold, the cardiologists, since they control the patients and were trained in coronary angiography, began taking over that procedure. Our referrals dwindled and we gave it up entirely. All coronary and heart catheterization work are done by cardiologists today. Cardiologists understand the physiology and pathology involved. We did our part in showing them how to place those groin catheters; they are basically the same ones used by Dr. Judkins back in the 1960s.

As the new technology became available, I think radiologists in northern Nevada kept pace. As things have progressed with the advent of cross-sectional imaging using ultrasound, CT scanning, PET, and MRI, we were, at best, only a half step behind the rest of the nation. Older radiologists spent a lot of time in conferences keeping abreast with continuing education and improved technology.

Endoscopies are popular these days. When you see Katie Couric on the *Today Show* having her colon "scoped" before twenty-five million people, you know this is going to be a popular procedure. We still do a limited number of GI exams on many of our senior patients who are in poor health, but we have different, modified techniques available to facilitate them. Endoscopies are quite good for most patients because bleeding ulcers can be cauterized and intestinal polyps can be removed. It has adjunctive status, but in a basic screening situation, the barium enema can still be very helpful for certain patients who would have problems with the scopes.

Liability Risk and Malpractice Insurance

From a medical-legal standpoint, radiology ranks fairly high in risk for malpractice, as reflected in high costs of liability insurance. The two procedures we do with the highest exposure risk are chest x-rays and mammograms. One would think highly invasive procedures would be the most risky because they are certainly the most complicated, but they have a fairly low liability. The basic day-to-day chest x-rays and mammograms done in great numbers are our most vulnerable procedures.

Studies have been done indicating that of a thousand chest films read by two peers in radiology, between 0.3 percent and 0.5 percent do not agree. Your average day-to-day radiologist, hopefully, is going to be that good. No one's perfect, and I think anybody who thinks he or she is perfect is living in a fantasy world.

I served continuously on the Washoe County Medical Society Medical-Legal Screening Panel for over thirty years and have learned much about that process. Having been a medical expert in this area, I know one should never be too cocky when entering the courtroom. You want to eat a bit of humble pie. Nevada used to have one of the best medical-legal screening systems in the nation, but the panel has been eliminated. Over the years, the panel filtered out as many as two-thirds of the cases that were frivolous. Panelists' findings would show there was no evidence of malpractice, and, subsequently, the suits would be dropped.

Lawyers got more aggressive over the years and were using these panels as fishing expeditions to gather information for a suit. So, it was finally concluded the panels had outlived their usefulness. For forty years, in two different formats, they were very effective advisory panels that began as volunteer groups of doctors and lawyers who would come together periodically to review cases of potential medical liability. After the panels were eliminated, they were briefly placed back into law and operated by the insurance division. Dr. Tom Brady was effective in having panel findings admissible in court and forcing attorneys to put up a bond for taking cases to court when the panel found no liability. That change was not enough; the panels were eventually eliminated.

Hospital Competition

One of the big turning points in the community was when Washoe Medical Center and St. Mary's Hospital decided to build new office buildings next to the hospital. Doctors who moved in learned the importance of having their offices next to the hospital. Some say doctor tenants were a "captive audience" of the hospital. Their being close just made their day much smoother by not having to drive back and forth to two or three different facilities. Surgeons and some of the subspecialties still have to be highly mobile because of the myriad of insurance and HMO policies. Office building were just one area the two hospitals competed.

There was a period when both major hospitals in town were vying to be the trauma center for the area, and the helicopter emergency service was the center of what was called the "Trauma Wars." I nicknamed the helicopters "medflies." I always thought it was better to have just one service rather than to compete for helicopter services. There was a lot of controversy over this issue. I thought there were times when bringing in a sick or injured patient might have been done faster by ambulance. The "medflies" add a layer of expense on medical care, but they serve a valuable purpose and are here to stay.

The designation of Washoe Medical Center as the area Trauma Center in the late 1980s was a good thing. In this day and age of subspecialization, there are people who are good at trauma work, such as, surgeons, orthopedists, and neurosurgeons. It is better for patients when subspecialties are under one roof and function as a team.

Managed Care

When managed care arrived in northern Nevada, it became a real problem. I was never very good as an administrator, and I considered myself a "pick and shovel" radiologist. I liked to be down in the pits doing the procedures and reading films. My shortcoming is in the business end of my practice. I have observed, over the years, that non-medical people were making medical decisions. This began in the mid-1960s with Medicare and Medicaid, and it has progressed steadily since then. Medicine started the change and the change has continued. Physicians in private practice find it difficult, having different payment schemes and certain percentages; they find it very frustrating as government and insurance companies eat away at their incomes. However, these agencies haven't found away to cover people without health insurance.

Health Insurance and Patients Health

I really don't know the answer to today's problem of millions upon millions of Americans not having health insurance. That's a sore point, and there just isn't much I can do about that. I know that my group never turned anybody away when they came into the emergency room without insurance. Did they lack preventive care because they didn't have proper insurance coverage? Probably, but by and large, there is healthcare for people in need. Just because they don't have some form of health insurance, does not mean they don't have access to healthcare.

I reflect, sometimes, on my experiences as a general practitioner in the early days of my career, and even then there were basically three influences that had a profound effect on my patients' health: smoking, drinking alcohol, and the wrong diet. These three factors are the toughest things to change.

People want a pill for this, a certain medical procedure for that, but they have no interest in changing their lifestyles. Exercise is not an option, they don't want to eat in moderation, they don't want to use alcohol in moderation, and they don't want to quit using tobacco products. Are they addicted to that lifestyle? I think they are. To narrow it down, I feel the most popular addiction, the one that kills and maims people by the millions each year is smoking. It is the simplest reversible risk factor that causes lung, heart, and vascular problems.

Oral cancers, with few exceptions, are attributed to the use of "smokeless tobacco." I see young boys trying to emulate baseball players with a wad of snuff, and they develop malignancies at an early age by using this chronic irritant. These individuals should step back two steps and listen to common sense about smoking, drinking, and eating. With moderation, many of the problems in American healthcare would be eliminated. There are a lot of other diseases that aren't directly caused by tobacco, but the majority of controllable diseases are self-determined.

Advances in Radiology

The specialty of radiology has spawned some interesting career fields and has provided opportunities for very valuable assistants and technicians. Radiology techs were being trained as long as forty-five years ago. They would assist with gastrointestinal work and do some of the basic bread-and-butter work. Then, as the profession became more advanced, the technologist portion also became much more advanced. As we started to "marry" the computer to the x-ray tube and to the old magnetic resonance device, things became complicated. Those of us who were near the end of our careers realized how much we depended on these finely-trained technologists. This became a very mutually beneficial situation. Just as radiologists pursued advanced training in one particular subspecialty or another, the same thing began occurring with the technicians. They have become very fine specialists in their own right. This is true with ultrasound techs, MRI techs, nuclear medicine techs, and all the other radiology subspecialty techs.

Radiation Oncologists

In recent years radiation oncologists, initially called radiation therapists, have come on the scene and actually do the implanting of prostate "seeds" that deliver radiation to the tumor. My daughter, Jenny, is a radiation oncologist and she works several times a week with urologists implanting isotopic "seeds." Patients have to be carefully evaluated before the "seeds" are implanted. Physicians have to look at the age and health of the patient; make comparisons with the other treatment modalities like external beam radiation or radical surgery; and then advise the patient on treatment. Overall statistics for all of these procedures are not that markedly different. There are some caveats with implantation, however. If the prostate specific antigen (PSA) test results start to rise after the "seeds" are implanted, the doctor sometimes wonders and worries if they were placed exactly in the right location.

It is also possible to treat prostatic cancer with external beam radiation with good results, and with either the external beam or the "seeds," the patient may eliminate surgery as an alternative. This decision is made after the urologist and the radiation oncologist go into excruciating detail about the various treatment options. Then, the patient can make an informed decision.

Scientists at the Lawrence laboratory in Berkeley, California, have developed artificial radioactive isotopes, an alternative to naturally occurring isotopes. They produce many artificial, short-lived isotopes, which are very useful. Isotope I_{131} is used in thyroid cancer therapy. Other such isotopes are used in diseases of liver, bone, lungs, kidneys, etc., and they are very effective. These isotopes weren't available during the years I trained.

The Future

What's coming down the pike in radiology? Well, we have a new generation of imaging devices, which are faster and make clearer images. The pixels become smaller, definition becomes greater, and pictures become much clearer. Medical researchers are also trying to minimize radiation exposure. One of the beneficial aspects of the MRI is that there is no x-ray exposure. It's just a great big magnetic field with molecular activation, which gives us a clearer picture. When the computer "marries" either the magnet or the CT scanner, the end product is magnificent images. The results of this technology shows improvement almost daily.

It's interesting that with all our new imaging technology and devices that produce excellent images, we are still looking at the same diseases, but in a much more finite way. MRI spectroscopy is effective in providing information on where specific drugs concentrate in the body. From this localization, doctors can refine dosage appropriateness for cancer of the heart and liver, for example. The CAT and MRI scanners are excellent diagnostic tools, and, in many instances, they help refine the definitive diagnosis, and differentiate between tumor and infection. They can provide information on whether or not the tumor has metastasized to the lungs or lymph nodes.

Retirement

At the time I retired, I was the only radiologist in my group who had not done a fellowship in some specific new imaging technology. Many of the procedures we did were getting very complicated, and even though I could hold my own doing the bread-and-butter work, the more recently-trained partners could do these procedures in addition to the newer more sophisticated procedures. I could see the "sunset" was just around the corner.

I can't estimate the exact number of radiologists in the area today, but every hospital in northern Nevada, including Carson City, has a number of well-trained, competent radiologists. I fit into the "dinosaur" class at this point. I retired in 1999, but after a year or so in retirement, I wasn't quite ready to turn in my number. Dr. Tom Barcia, chief of staff at the Veterans Administration Medical Center, called and asked if I would come over and read a few films. That was a little over two years ago, and it occurs to me that I am like an aluminum can—I am being "recycled!" Do I enjoy it? You bet. Many of the University of Nevada medical students rotate through the VA and there are excellent training programs at the VA. There are three to five students in each radiology rotation, and I find it warming and stimulating to teach. We have a number of excellent tools for doing day-to-day, "bread-and-butter," radiology at the VA, and it seems to still be a hand-in-glove arrangement for me at this point.

While I was busy with my practice and doing community and professional work, there seemed to be enough time to raise a wonderful family. Jeanne and I have four children—three elected to have a career in medicine: Eric is an orthopedist, Jenny is a radiation oncologist, and Scott just returned to Reno a year ago as an oral surgeon. My fourth child, John, decided to go into law and is also practicing in Reno. Jeanne and I haven't decided if we created a tribe or a hazard; it is hard to know at this time. I was director of the YMCA early morning "Fitness Class" for twenty-five years, and I was chairman of the Physicians Aid Committee from its inception in 1981. Hopefully, my legacy will be felt in the area for many years to come—long after my passing. It has been a great and rewarding career and I would not have changed a thing.

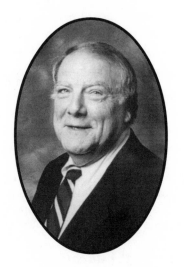

Dr. Wesley Hall

16: Dr. Wesley Hall, Surgery

Early Life

I was born in Memphis, Tennessee, on July 29, 1939. I grew up in Shelby, Mississippi, a small town that had more cotton gins than any other town in the world. I went to high school there, and I went to "Old Miss" for two years, but, as a result of my father moving to Reno during the World War II, I came to Reno to finish my last year of undergraduate work at the University of Nevada. I came to Nevada before Interstate 80 was built. I remember crossing Utah on "old" Highway 40 and coming into Nevada; every time a road took off in the desert there was a big yellow sign with black lettering saying, "Warning, no food, gas, or water for the next one hundred miles." I thought, "Now that's my kind of country."

There was a long line of physicians in my family and each was Wesley W. Hall, M.D., but none was a junior or whatever, as our middle names were different. My father, grandfather, and great grandfather were all doctors. Even my great-great grandfather practiced medicine although he would be called a "preceptor," a man who "studied" medicine under another doctor due to the scarcity of medical schools during his time.[1]

Dr. Robert Hollingsworth came to Shelby in the mid 1940s and took over the Hall Clinic and Hospital, which my grandfather and uncle had built. As a little fellow, I remember that back in the operating room was a closet and a big autoclave for sterilizing things. Dr. Hollingsworth, who retired a couple of years ago and was about ninety, called me one day to say he was getting some of his stuff and looking around, and that he had suspected that the closet had not been opened for at least fifty years. He opened the creaky door and found some old books and things. He said he was going to send me one of the books after he had read it. It was written by Dr. Wesley W. Hall and was titled, *"Dyspepsia,"* published in 1877. Here was a book written by my great grandfather. One of the funny things written was about halitosis. He wrote that halitosis was obviously caused by eating too much meat. "Meat sours in your stomach." he wrote. "You know, if you are going along the road now on a hot summer day and this dead dog is down on the side of the road, the stench comes up and it's because the meat has putrefied. That's where halitosis comes from. You eat meat and it putrefies in your stomach." Dr. Hollingsworth sent me the book and I found some other unusual ideas in it. One day I might donate that book to the History of Medicine program.

Medical Education

I have lots of memories such as this from growing up, and there was never a doubt that I, too, would be a physician. I finished my premed courses at the University of Nevada and Old Miss. I hated to leave "my kind of country," but I went to medical school there since there was no medical school in Nevada at the time.

After medical school, I did an internship in Denver before doing a two-year stint in the navy. I always thought of becoming a surgeon. There was no doubt as I always needed to see results, and to see folks get well. Surgery is dynamic and I liked that part of it.

I completed my surgical residency in Denver at the University of Colorado after my military service. Colorado, at that time, was one of the "hot spots" for surgical training and there were a number of outstanding physicians there doing transplant work. One of Colorado's strengths was their excellent program, which pioneered kidney transplants. It was such a great program that I actually considered staying in Denver, but Denver was exploding with growth, and my father needed somebody to go in with him, so I was drawn back to Nevada.

Surgery in Reno

The Move to Reno

The year was 1971 when I set up my practice in Reno, and things were noticeably different from today. There were no central venous catheters being placed in patients in Reno and, especially, there was no hyper-alimentation being done. As I had been trained to do these things in

Denver, I brought these procedures to Reno. I went to the local pharmacies in town and had them begin stocking hyperalimentation solutions, such as, "Dr. Hall's number one," and "Dr. Hall's number two." That was the beginning of hyperalimentation in Reno.

The number of surgeons in town had been stable for many years, and they were a very good group. When I arrived, in addition to my father, there were Drs. Kenneth Maclean, Bill Tappan, Bob Simon, Warren McClellan, Donald Guisto, John Sande, Gilbert Lenz, Bill Dane, Fred Anderson and a few others, and that was pretty much the surgery team here. It was a relatively small group that expanded rapidly after I came. Then, as now, there was never a shortage of general surgeons in Reno and, as new surgical technologies and procedures were developed in the early 1980s, the practice of surgery and Reno's population really took off.

The MGM Grand Hotel and Casino was built later in the 1970s and four or five other casinos sprang up. Anne, whom I had married in 1961 when she was a graduate student at George Washington University, commented after a few years in town, "Oh, Reno isn't going to grow, it's just going to explode," and I said, "No, it can't because there isn't enough water here for any more people." She was right in the short term, but I think in the long term, I will be proven right. We don't have enough water for all these people. Recently, area planners reported that water might run out by the year 2020.

Since Reno is such a nice place to live, doctors have been attracted from all parts of the country to set up practices here. This influx of doctors has created an enviable physician/patient ratio—much better than Las Vegas or many other places in the country.

With all the changes in insurance programs taking place today, it seems insignificant that one of the first changes catching my attention was insurance companies requiring patients to be admitted to the hospital the morning of their surgery rather than the night before. I thought all my patients would balk at this, but they did not. Not a peep. This policy change went through like goose grease, and, in looking back, this may well have been the beginning of what today is called "managed care."

In the mid 1980s as new technology and new surgical procedures came on the scene, the cost of medical care began to soar. Then the managed care people used this as a reason to bring on the diminution of individual physician's input and control concerning treatment of patients, and this continues today.

I'm not sure many physicians in town saw this coming; I didn't. It sort of crept up on us. This erosion of our profession was happening more in other areas of the country than here, due our isolation, but

Reno is an interesting place because of this isolation. It is a long way to big population centers, and the population here hasn't always been large enough for insurance companies to battle each other over getting "market share" because there wasn't that big of a market share to be had here.

Before I came to town, I had met several surgeons: Gilbert Lenz, John Sande, and Ken Maclean, and I liked them all. There seemed to be much more camaraderie among all the doctors than what we have today. Maybe it's me, but I feel there is more competition for patients now than in the early days of my practice. Maybe it's the managed care aspect, the business aspect of the practice of medicine, that is causing this. Patients have lost decision-making ability in their choice of doctor, their choice of hospital, their choice of medications, and they are the real losers in this competitive marketplace.

When I came to town, St. Mary's did not keep its emergency room open at night. The hospital closed up and you could ring the doorbell and one of the Sisters would come down to see what was the problem. At that time my office was right across the street from St. Mary's; many times I thought to myself, I couldn't practice in a hospital where I couldn't get an x-ray or lab work in the middle of the night. So, Dr. Mike Gainey and I decided we would push for keeping the ER open at night. Mike was a general surgeon who had come to town at the same time as me and who shared an office with me. As a result of our inquiry, St. Mary's opened an all-night ER, and we had to man it for quite a while until the hospital hired Dr. Paul White to staff it. We had full practices during the day and staffed the ER at night, but we were much younger in those days.

At that time Washoe had a fully-equipped emergency room open around the clock, but it did not have full-time physician staffing. There seemed to always be one or two doctors around, and they would call in specialists as needed: like for delivering a baby, stitching up lacerations, or treating pneumonia. Physician participation in those emergency rooms during this time was much greater as hospitals began hiring emergency medical specialists. Also, large numbers of the population were not using the emergency rooms as their primary care facilities either.

I got to know administrators pretty well in those early days and was most impressed with the foresightedness of Sister Seraphine at St. Mary's Hospital. At that time St. Mary's was not the number one hospital in town, and Sister Seraphine saw the need to expand; the hospital had ample funds to build more and bigger facilities than they actually needed at the time. She saw construction costs rising and she had the foresight to build several extra floors into which they gradually expanded.

The administrator at Washoe was Carroll Ogren, and it was no secret that Carroll had his bouts with alcohol from time to time, but he was a better administrator when he was drinking than most were when cold sober. Carroll knew all the employees at Washoe by their first names. He knew them all. He didn't have to use "time and motion studies" before making important decisions. I remember one morning going into his office and telling him, "You know, you're losing money because I can't get my cases scheduled in your operating rooms. I might have to even turn them over to St. Mary's." That was a Thursday morning about ten o'clock. The following Monday morning at seven-thirty he had two new ORs open with complete staff hired and ready to go.

I'm not sure, but I think when Sister Seraphine at St. Mary's turned "about one hundred years old," she was replaced by Bud Reveley who wanted St. Mary's to be "all things" to "all people" and had big ideas. Well, his big ideas were to make a mark and to move on to a bigger hospital someplace. Before he was "forced out," Bud started the hospital on a path that probably should have been "treaded on" with a bit more hesitancy. The hospital made some mistakes early on, and gradually the nuns who were running the place got eased out of the front office and replaced with the guys with sharp pencils behind their ears, the "bean counters."

As new medical technology and equipment were being created and developed elsewhere, such as CT scanners, hospital administrators began taking a keen interest in "bottom line." Health planners on the state level, however, were reluctant to allow healthcare providers and others to purchase such expensive equipment because they were concerned that healthcare costs would get out of hand quickly if equipment was duplicated at every facility in the state. A Certificate of Need program was initiated, and I got involved in that somewhat.

Because doctors were busy taking care of sick folks and weren't paying attention to what was going on in hospital administration and on the government level, we quickly got behind the eight ball without realizing it. There was also a big push to decrease the number of patients admitted to acute care hospitals and, once admitted, to get them out faster and faster. This cost containment interest by insurers contributed to the rise of outpatient surgical facilities in a big way.

Surgeons became concerned that their patients might be rushed out of the acute care settings too fast. We can't make things heal any faster than God does. We can't take somebody who is seventy years old with diabetes and all kinds of problems and do a colon resection on them and get them out of the hospital in four days. They just don't get well that quickly. This "cost containment at any cost" mentality has always been a sore point with me. I have always maintained that the "best" medical care in the world will be the "least expensive" medical care in the world in the long run.

It seems that governments periodically get infatuated with ill-conceived healthcare concepts. Take Diagnosis Related Groups (DRGS), Certificates of Need regulations, Professional Standards Review Organizations (PSROS) for examples. All of these were cost containment concepts that were ineffective and faded away after a time.

There are "pencil pushers" who figure the doctor can reduce length of stay in the hospital, if there are cuts here and trimming there. They reason that the bottom line is improved if the workforce is reduced, and the lists go on and on. After a while, there is no more trimming possible, and they have to face the fact that quality healthcare will continue to be expensive.

Advances in Surgery

There have been dramatic advances in surgery over the last thirty years, such as new instrumentation, procedures, diagnostic test, imaging equipment, antibiotics, and other excellent drugs, but the thing to remember is that with any invasive procedure, it is the surgeon who has to do the procedure. Today, physicians have basically the same hand-eye coordination and reflexes they had years and years ago, and it will be the same in future years. The surgeon's skills at doing things with his or her hands cannot exponentially improve; however, one of the major technological advances and one that has tested hand-eye coordination to the maximum is the introduction of the laparoscope. It has replaced many traditional surgical techniques and is the "preferred" technique for many procedures, such as gall bladder removal. Now, ninety-nine percent of the time the gall bladder can be removed in this manner, but sometimes, if something is not quite right, it just can't be done. When that happens, rather than going home the same day, the patient has to stay in the hospital for three to five days. Insurance companies hate when that happens.

Vascular Surgery

My special interest has always been in peripheral vascular surgery, and there have been a number of improvements in this area over the years. Although I do not do heart surgery, I have seen angioplasty technology dramatically improve the patient's outcome. The placement and expansion of those small balloons and stents continue to be effective in opening blocked blood vessels without the need for major invasive procedures. This is always a benefit to patients.

We will have to continually work for methods and mechanisms

that will hold those vessels open, as they are prone to clogging up again. Work is being done to construct "super stents" that resist this clogging process, but changes in this area of medicine will be slow, and dramatic progress may not be available tomorrow. No matter how far we advance, people are going to die. We can't keep them alive forever. We just try to maintain a good quality of life for the years they have left.

Diseases

The diseases and health conditions physicians are treating today are the same ones we have been treating for years, but I think we are making progress in finding them earlier. One of the things that distresses me is that medical students don't rely nearly as much on physical examinations and observations as they should. I've talked with students and have found many of them will quickly recommend use of technology and testing to help make their diagnoses. That is the first thing they think about, rather than doing a hands-on examination—seeing where the tenderness is—listening to the patient. They start ordering tests. It's true that imaging technology has advanced today and provides very valuable information, but you still can't beat that personal touch in making your diagnosis.

Antibiotics

We have had major advances in antibiotics and these have played a big role in advancing surgery, but the big bug-a-boo is still the infection. The more we use antibiotics, the more we're finding that some of the "bugs" are becoming resistant to them.

A number of physicians have the tendency to prescribe a new broad-spectrum antibiotic, and they treat everything with it without good indication. Soon they get resistant organisms and then look for the newer drugs and use them in the same way, and the cycle continues.

Pneumonia is still one of the major worries of surgeons today, especially if patients have other problems, such as diabetes, heart trouble, kidney failure, or other illnesses. Sadly enough, many surgeons consider pneumonia as the "friend of the aged," and it still takes its toll on the aged.

Cancer

When I came to town, there were no oncologists and I had to do a lot of cancer treatment on my surgical patients. Patients who needed chemotherapy had very few agents available to them. One of the drugs I used frequently was Fluorouracil (5 FU), and it was as good as any available. I didn't know exactly how much to give them. I would bring them in the hospital and push the 5 FU on them until their blood count started falling, until it started suppressing their bone marrow, and then I would back off. That was about the only drug to use. There were not many effective treatments and very few cures; I just tried to control the cancer as much as I could. Many times, I tired to make the time they had left the best possible. Chemotherapy, in those who could tolerate it, made patients quite sick, and the quality of their lives was not very good. I often wondered if they wouldn't be better off with a bottle of bourbon and a fishing pole.

The big breakthroughs in medicine, not just surgery, are going to be in pharmacology, genetics, and being able to develop vaccines and treatments for diseases that we can't even envision now. I feel there will be no big breakthroughs in surgery or cardiology in the very near future. There will be little advances—the surgical techniques will improve and better instruments may come along, but wherever humans have to do things with their hands, there are not going to be quantum leaps.

In my field of surgery like in other specialties, there are few diseases that can be prevented. A hernia develops due to defects and appendicitis just happens. I don't know of a lot of ways to prevent them. Some other conditions, such as lung and colon cancers, do lend themselves to prevention and steps can be taken to decrease frequency.

Breast Cancer

I have often wondered whether all the hormones we've given women over the last thirty to forty years have been instrumental in increasing incidences of breast cancer and, if so, whether preventative measures can be taken. In the mid 1960s the incidence of breast cancern in the nation was about 1 in 12 women and then along came birth control pills. The incidence of hormone distribution among young women went sky high and then a few years later came a rise in the incidence of breast cancer. Now that incidence is about 1 in 8.7, which is a big jump for one disease.

Today there is a lot of discussion on what is the best surgical method of removing tumors in the breast. I have always felt that the best way to cure cancer is to take it out and put it in a jar somewhere. I think years ago the dictum in surgery was "If it's a big cancer, do a little operation, biopsy it, but if it is a little cancer, get that thing out!" The basic principle was to make wide margins and locate normal tissue to get around the cancer. There are some selective patients where a quadrantectomy, which is a removal of part of the breast with axillary lymph node radiation, gives as good a result as a mastectomy, but these women are committed to perhaps six weeks of radiation. If they are from Tonopah or Pioche or somewhere else out of town, it is difficult for them to get in to do that. Then, I always wonder, "Did I get it all?" I have kept a record of all the patients I have operated on for breast cancer since I went into practice, and I think that the cure rate is better than *Ladies Home Journal* and the *Reader's Digest* indicate. Tons of literature about breast cancer is available and there is no shortage of people writing books about how to manage it.

I think there are two absolute contraindications to doing a lumpectomy for breast cancer: if the tumor is more than two centimeters in size, or if it is real close to the nipple. The surgeon can't get far enough around these tumors. In addition, some women have small bosoms, which cosmetically doesn't lend itself to a quadrantectomy procedure. They would be much better off with a mastectomy with reconstructive surgery.

I think the cure rate for breast cancer has been improving and is very good today if surgeons get it the first time around. My recommendation to my patients has always been not to "pluck around on it," but to go in and give it the very best shot; shoot the big gun at that time.

I've had one-half dozen women over the years that wanted to have a lumpectomy. They were quite concerned about losing their breast, and I've said, "Well, I can't do a lumpectomy but I will refer you to somebody who will." They went to somebody else in town and had their lumpectomy. Three of those came back to me within eighteen months with a recurrence of their cancers. Two of them did well, but one did not. I didn't think they should have had lumpectomies.

New surgeons coming to town prefer to leave that decision entirely up to their patients, but I have always felt that I have to look at myself in the mirror shaving every morning and I don't want to wonder if I am doing something I don't think is right.

Occasionally, my patients ask about alternative treatment for this or that, and my only advice is if it works for you, so be it. Testimonials on different over-the-counter (OTC) cures are hard to prove or disprove, and I have said, "It's hard to argue with success." Herbal medications and copper bracelets make some people feel better. I say, "Well, good for them." The problem with a lot of those OTC cures is that if somebody has a curable illness that can be caught early, but treatment is postponed by trying these various things, that's where the big danger comes. It's hard to believe people can be really harmed by taking St. John's Wort or Ginkgo biloba, to name a few. There are so many different kinds of natural drugs and therapies people will grasp at if they get desperate, or if they think they can be made to look or act younger or live longer.

Health Style and Weight Reduction

Over the years it seems that the best advice a doctor could ever give his patients would be to exercise. There is no question that people who exercise have fewer problems than those who are sedentary and those who do not watch their weight or diet. I mean, your mamma told you that. You never want to pork up like a sow going to slaughter.

My overweight patients ask me if they might be candidates for stapling their stomachs, but I always advise them that procedure has all the makings of a crutch. Stapling does not last forever and frequently the staples come undone, but it seems to be effective for a lot of people, at least initially. It helps some people, and I don't remember what the numbers are, but if you take one hundred obese people and staple their stomachs, in two years seventy-five or eighty of them are going to be up to their pre-op weight. Through stretching and having the staples pull through, they eat their way through it.

A procedure that was popular when I was a resident was the jejunal by-pass surgery. I remember an attorney's wife in Denver had this procedure done and she had all kinds of mental problems as a result. I remember her surgeon lamented the fact that he had done it. She called him one night and said if he didn't hook her back up right now, she was going to blow her brains out. They went back in, reversed her intestinal bypass, and, not surprisingly, in a couple of months her weight was back up to where she was before. She didn't blow her brains out.

Organized Medicine

As most people know, my father, Wesley W. Hall, M.D., was the president of the American Medical Association, and I am frequently asked if I have interest in going in that direction in organized medicine. I usually tell them that having one AMA president in the family is quite enough. I got turned off to organized medicine a good while ago when the Nevada State Medical Association held its annual meeting in Elko one year and the pilot who was to take the Las Vegas delegation home got drunk and couldn't fly the chartered plane. That held them up a day or so, and as a result, they pushed through a policy that future meetings could only be in Reno or Las Vegas, or within fifty miles of the airports in those cities. That was something I strongly disagreed with as it eliminated holding annual meetings in the fun places like Ely and Elko that seriously relied on convention business. That thinking effectively eliminated me from further service in organized medicine.

I did serve as chief of staff at Washoe Medical Center for two years and let it be known up front that I thought doctors ought to have a major say in how the hospital was run. It was a losing battle. Hospitals today have gotten to be such a big business, and physicians are less and less important cogs in the administrative wheel than they ever were.

One of the first things I was confronted with as chief of staff was the fact that the entire pathology department was to be replaced with another outfit. The administrator expected a rubber stamp approval from me of this policy change. His notion was that I worked for him, and I had to tell him that I didn't see it that way at all. I felt he was working for me and he had overstepped his bounds.[2]

Being hospital chief of staff, in years past, was a responsibility doctors took on when there wasn't much for them to do. The medical staffs were small and there was a lot of physician cooperation. With the diversification of medical specialties and the increase in the number of staff members, a need was created to have some kind of central control and somebody to oversee it; that guy was called the chief of staff. He was the one who saw to it that doctors who practiced in the hospital worked according to the bylaws. Many doctors simply don't want to do that and somebody has to be the sergeant-of-arms. It has to be that way. My take on it was that I was the physicians' advocate and as long as they were doing things in a reasonable manner, that was fine; there could be no intimidation of employees, no gross negligence, and doctors must behave as ladies and gentlemen.

I enjoyed those two years as chief of staff, and they were eye openers for me. Since then I have enjoyed my work in Reno, raising and educating my children, getting them married off, and welcoming my three grandchildren into the family. My half-brother is a career military physician, and my son recently returned to Reno after being educated in the art and science of plastic and reconstructive surgery. He is the fifth Wesley W. Hall, M.D.,. in the Hall medical "dynasty."

A Heck of a Place to Live

Reno has been one heck of a place to live and raise my family, and I have enjoyed the medical community immensely. I relocated my family to North Carolina for a few years in the 1980s, but we were happy to return to the Silver State, as I like the hunting, camping, and fishing. My wife, Anne, and I enjoy the many friendships we have made over the years. I plan to continue to practice and, as I tell my colleagues who ask me, "When are you going to retire?" I will always say, "I will retire two years after I die."

Notes

[1] This was a common way to become a physician before 1900. No formal education was required.

[2] Administrator Robert Burn negotiated with another group of pathologists and tried to replace the existing group. Dr. Wes Hall and the executive committee of the hospital forced him to give the contract to the existing group led by Drs. Roger Ritzlin and Anton Sohn.

17: Dr. Joseph Reinkemeyer, Urology

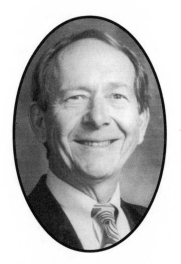

Dr. Joseph Reinkemeyer

Early Life

I was born March 3, 1935, and raised in Rich Fountain, Missouri. My family owned a dairy farm, and I lived on the farm until I entered college. My father borrowed money to buy the farm in 1927. He was a self-taught veterinarian—later becoming a county judge and a realtor in order to survive the Great Depression. Although he needed a license to practice veterinary medicine and was warned about doing it without one, he still helped out with all the neighbors' livestock.

I had orthopedic problems with my feet, and people at the local vocational center did not encourage me to go to medical school with such impairment. However my grades were quite good and after high school I chose to go to Missouri University. When my father found out about my interest in the university, he said, "No, if you are going to go to college, it will be at St. Louis University." It is a Jesuit school that was held in high esteem. There were 240 students in my premed class, but after four years, only eighteen of us were accepted into medical school.

There were no physicians in my family, but due to my feet problems and subsequent surgeries, I became a good friend with Dr. Ossman, who was from Jefferson City. He frequently came down to the farm to go rabbit hunting, and when I was eight or nine years old, I kenneled his hunting dogs. One time I had twenty-three beagles running in unison in those Missouri hills.

Dr. Ossman was a real great guy and fine general surgeon. On many of his visits, he brought politicians and other dignitaries from the city. I admired him a lot and he encouraged my interest in a medical career. That was my only association with a physician, but my mom's sister was a nurse and a nun and would give us special care at the hospital in Jefferson City on my frequent visits.

A Career in Medicine and Urology

I went through undergraduate and premed at St. Louis and then went on to medical school, finishing in 1961. I took a straight medical internship at the St. Louis University Hospital. I had developed an interest in urology, and I did the required year of general surgery at the Jewish hospital in St. Louis. Following that, I completed my urology residency at Barnes Hospital, Washington University in St. Louis.

The physician draft was going on during medical school. In order to get a decent residency, I had to either have completed military service or be in the Berry Plan, which would defer me during my residency. I would then be allowed to practice my specialty in the military, giving me more options. I went through the whole list of specialties and alphabetically the last one, of course, was urology. Just to make my decision simple, I thought, "You know, that's not a bad idea."

The other thought I had was that if I couldn't stand on my feet for long periods and wanted a surgical practice, I could at least sit and do a transurethral resections of the prostate (TURP) and similar procedures. That is essentially how I chose urology.

When I was in my residency, renal transplantation was just coming into vogue, as was renal angiography. We did angiograms, threading catheters, and translumbar injections into the aorta right above the renal artery to outline the kidneys. To determine if a renal mass was malignant, we needed as much information as possible and angiograms provided that information. It was still a relatively crude procedure and had a fair amount of morbidity associated with it. It was like the old carotid angiograms, in which a needle was inserted into the carotid artery causing the patient a lot of discomfort. Another procedure, the intravenous pyelogram (IVP) was also well established at that time.

Where I trained was an impressive bladder cancer treatment program using a urinary diversion technique developed by Dr. Eugene Bricker. Barnes Hospital was a leader in treating bladder cancer. Cervical cancers were treated with radon implants, external beam radiation, and parametrial gold. That treatment sometimes resulted in bladder and colon fistulas, and Bricker allowed us to treat these complications.

I really enjoyed my training at Washington University and Barnes Hospital and actually considered going into practice with one of the staff urologists there named Robert Royce, a good friend and a marvelous fellow.

Urology in Reno

The Move to Reno

My civilian consultant at Travis Air Force Base, Dr. Bill Smart, told me there was good opportunity in the Reno area for a urologic surgeon. After meeting with Dr. Hoyt Miles, who was practicing urology in Reno, I fell in love with the place. I had only intended to "kick around Reno" for a year or two before going back to St. Louis. Drs. Hoyt Miles, Carl Sauls, Joe Tuttle, Jake Detar, and Gordy Nitz were the only urology men in town in 1968, and I decided my friend was right, there was excellent opportunity here.

I really think that by 1971 or 1972, our medical community in Reno didn't take second seat to any other medical community in the country. It was really that good. When I came to town, I started to do my own arteriograms, but then I met Dr. Fred Boyden, who had come to town a year earlier. He was a real solid, substantial radiologist, and a credit to the community.

I always referred patients who needed radiologic studies out of my office, mainly because I didn't want anyone saying, "You did the IVP because you had a financial incentive for doing it." I never did set up x-ray equipment in my office. It's known that for every one thousand IVPs, one is going to get a very serious untoward reaction. I just felt that if there is no financial incentive and if one has an adequate medical indication for ordering the film, one would be in good shape for any criticism. We had very good radiologists in Reno. Another excellent radiologists came to town, Dr. Fred Stahl, who was another plus for the community. Fred was one of the first radiologists to do x-rays outside of the hospital setting in Reno.

Washoe Medical Center

I have always enjoyed working at Washoe Medical Center, the county hospital at the time, and I particularly enjoyed working with the administrator, Carroll Ogren. Sometimes Carroll had to be begged to order new equipment for the urology department, but somehow he always got it for us. I favored Washoe in those days, admitting most of my patients there, as it was more of a twenty-four hour hospital than St. Mary's. Even at well-run Washoe, there were interesting medical stories to tell. It seems there has always been a nursing shortage, so I would advise my patients, " If you can't get anyone to help you and you're having a real problem during the night, just call 9-1-1." So, one night a patient calls 9-1-1 and the operator says, "What's wrong?" The patient says, "I'm bleeding to death!" "Well, where are you?" "I'm in room 309 at Washoe Hospital." The dispatcher then called the nursing supervisor on the third floor and that patient got a nurse within three minutes. It worked really well.

Bladder Cancer

It's interesting that the incidence of bladder cancer hasn't changed all that much since I came to Reno. I trained at a major center for bladder cancer, and we were inundated with it. In those days, too, when people had blood in the urine, the physician would give them an antibiotic, and the bleeding would stop. Then six months or a year later they would have blood again and, by then, they would have a large tumor mass in their bladder.

Kidney Transplants

We don't do kidney transplants in northern Nevada, but we harvested quite a few for out of state transplanting at centers. My colleagues, Drs. Dave Johnson and Paul Clark, who were nephrologists, were so very good at talking to families and next of kin in getting permission for organ donations. We took care of a large Native American population, and they traditionally have a high incidence of diabetes with renal disease. Many of them required a kidney transplant. During the 1970s and early 1980s, we harvested more kidneys, per capita, than anyplace else in the United States. I would harvest kidneys and fly them in my plane, usually at night, to San Francisco or occasionally to University of California, Davis Medical Center in Sacramento, California.

It wasn't long before the "Federalies" got involved with the transplant program and mandated that all harvested organs go through organ donor centers. It seemed our northern Nevada patients awaiting transplants of the organs we harvested and delivered got priority on those organs. We always thought that was just great for "our" patients waiting for kidneys, but "not so" said the "Feds." Since our program in Reno was curtailed, Drs. Johnson and Clark were virtually out of the loop of organ procurement.

Kidney Stones

One thing that has really changed tremendously over the years has been the management of kidney stones. We would see a patient, who was very sick, septic with a complicated infection and a stone stuck in their ureter. I had to operate on them right away no matter the time or the day, or I would run the risk of losing them. Now with the new methods of percutaneous renal drainage, improved endoscopic access, and excellent antibiotics, great strides have been made. We still use instruments to go up into the ureters to take out stones that won't pass, which has been a big advantage and comfort for the patient.

The first stone unit, the lithotriptor, was brought to the South Bay in northern California by two urologists from Stanford medical school, and I must say, I was greatly impressed with this new technology. Next came a mobile unit, but there was concern about possible breakdown of that sophisticated equipment due to hauling it all over the western United States. It worked quite well, however, and it was fairly easy to learn how to use it. The first lithotriptors were bulky. The patient had to be submerged in water, but the newer ones used a gel and water bags, and that made things a lot better. There was experimentation using the lithotriptor to crush gallstones, but it just didn't seem to work that well.

Prostate Cancer

Endoscopic surgery for prostate cancer is replacing many open procedures, and it's ironic that the first endoscopic procedure was the TURP. It has been done for many years and is quite commonplace, but now, since it requires hospitalization, the Medicare program will no longer reimburse physicians adequately for it, so fewer and fewer are being done. Thermal therapy has virtually replaced the TURP; it is done in the physician's office and Medicare reimbursement is much better. It does keep the patient out of the expensive hospital and shrinking Medicare reimbursement became a disincentive for doctors doing them in the hospital. Young doctors coming out of residencies only do five or ten TURPs during their training that it is probably only safe for them to do a TURP on a small prostate gland. Also, drugs have made surgery for benign prostatic hypertrophy (BPH) less necessary.

Where I trained we did digital rectal exams on just about all men over fifty years old, and if there was a bump, lump, or hardness, we would biopsy the prostate. It would be done in a hospital under general anesthesia and patients would be admitted the night before surgery. We would use larger needles then and take more cores than today. It was much more of a production than biopsy procedures today.

Early in my career, I would go over to the hospital to see my patients the night before and then usually the next afternoon or the following morning they would go home. In those days, if I wanted to do an IVP on a patient, the patient would request, "Well, you have to admit me to the hospital because then my insurance will cover it." So, I would sit there and inform them, "It's going to cost you more to go into the hospital even though your insurance will pay for it because you will have to come up with money after the deductible is covered by the insurance company. It will definitely cost you less if you go to a radiologist's office and have it done." But most of them wouldn't hear of that and if I insisted on it, they would find another doctor who would put them in the hospital to do it.

There have been many improvements in prostate surgery over the years. In the days before antibiotics, the surgery of choice was called the perineal prostatectomy, and it was the only way to remove an enlarged prostate. These glands were often infected and outcomes were, many times, not very good; patients frequently died. Usually, after surgery we had to put in drainage tubes into the bladder and leave them in place for up to four weeks. On removing them, the incision would eventually heal and the patient could urinate again.

When I first started practice, people who had prostate nodules suspicious for cancer and had trouble passing urine were candidates for biopsy. If a cancer was found, we would do a radical perineal prostatectomy. The advantage, of course, in going perineally rather than via the suprapubic route was that an abdominal incision wasn't necessary; therefore, morbidity and recovery time were less. Bleeding was much less also, and, with the advances in antibiotic therapy, the use of drainage tubes in the bladder and urethra was reduced.

Erectile Dysfunction

I want to cover another subject that has really changed over the years, and that is the treatment for erectile dysfunction (ED). Back in the 1960s and during my residency, the first thing we looked for in people with ED was diabetes, and I can probably count five or six young men I diagnosed with diabetes simply because they came in to talk about their erectile dysfunction. Diabetes was one of the diseases that could go otherwise unrecognized and could cause erectile dysfunction. In those days people with impotence were thought to have psychosomatic problems. They go out and get swacked with booze, go home and try to have sex, and when they fail, they blame it on being tired or having had too much to drink. The next time they try and fail they start worrying, and worry is just about all it takes to increase the dysfunction. Hypertension, vascular disease, and their treatment, can be a leading factor in ED also.

In the early days of ED I would put in penile implants, but before I would do that, I would refer my patients to Dr. Ira Pauly at the University of Nevada School of Medicine for a psychological screen. There is nothing worse than to implant that equipment in someone who really didn't need it. A nightmare would be to have a patient return to me saying, "You ruined my life forever because I've got this rod in there and I did not need it." In thinking back, I probably implanted a fair amount of penile prostheses, when some patients would have been excellent candidates for Viagra, were it available then.

There is a drug called Yohimbine that shows effectiveness in probably twenty to twenty-five percent of the people with ED. In the early days it was combined with a small amount of strychnine, which evidently facilitated neurotransmission. Now the strychnine has been removed and you can buy Yohimbine over the counter.

For a while, penile injections as a treatment for ED became very popular. We would inject various substances directly into the penis and that would alleviate the problem. It was satisfactory for quite a few of my patients, mainly those who only infrequently had intercourse. It worked out very well for them. On following those patients for a while, they kind of dropped out and I think having sex became less important for them and the injections diminished.

When Viagra came along and the drug companies were good enough to give us samples, anybody who had a problem and wasn't on nitroglycerin would give it a try, and a lot of people were very pleased with it. I think it does enjoy a good amount of popularity and utilization.

Advances in Urology

The drug advances for the specialty of urology have been nothing less than spectacular. The anticancer drug, cisplatinum, came into use in the late 1960s and a totally new generation of chemotherapy was introduced. Up until that time, patients with germ cell testicle cancers, such as the kind cyclist Lance Armstrong had, didn't fare so well. Only about twenty percent of them survived and these were typically young men between eighteen and thirty years old. Today, irrespective of how advanced their disease, probably ninety percent of patients are cured with a combination of chemotherapy and surgery.

There is a philosophy now of "watchful waiting" because we have excellent imaging technology available. In the old days, we really had no equipment that would give us an idea what was going on with the lymph nodes without actually going in and taking a biopsy. Today we have such excellent scanning technology available, such as computerized axial tomography, magnetic resonance imaging, and ultrasound that we can see into every area of the body, and this has led to differing philosophies regarding treatment choices. Today we can "wait and see" while carefully following our patients as frequently as every three months. Not all doctors, however, feel this way.

I think many urologic cancers have such a wide biological spectrum; some fit the criteria for a cancer diagnosis, but are very slow growing, and others are just totally wild and aggressive. Prostate cancer is unique in that we have a fairly good handle on grading the cancer. We have a "Gleason Score," a one to ten rating based on the microscopic morphology of the cells. The cells are graded on the architecture and how malignant they look. In a urologist's practice, the Gleason Score is an excellent and remarkable tool in judging the aggressiveness of the cancer, thereby directing treatment.

The prostate specific antigen (PSA) is another test that provides important information about prostate cancer. If we remove a cancerous prostate, the PSA test, in most cases, reverts to negative, so it is a very valuable technology and has been just a great, great tool for urologists to follow their patients after treatment. There are a couple of small, non-prostate glands in the body that actually make a little PSA, so if someone has a very low level detectable PSA, it may not indicate that the cancer has returned.

In diagnosing prostate cancer, a major consideration is the age of the patient. Dr. Thomas Stamey, one of the nation's leading authorities on prostate cancer, has said, "I wouldn't do a radical prostatectomy on any patient over eighty unless he came in with his father." Basically, I wouldn't have considered doing surgery on patients over seventy. I felt that at seventy, one could get ten years with minimal amount of hassle and morbidity without the added potential morbidity of surgery. That was sort of my criteria. There were a few exceptions, but I would say that ninety percent of all my radical prostatectomy patients were under the age of seventy.

Of the three options urologists have in treating prostate cancer (surgery, chemotherapy, and radiation), and if all things are equal, I think surgery would serve the patient best, especially for men under sixty-five years old. Radiation in any form carries a long-term downside, and if someone has an isolated nodule, radiation seeds will probably have as good of a result as surgery, and morbidity is less.

I also think conformal radiation treatment is reasonably effective for someone over seventy who has an aggressive tumor. I like it even better than implanting radioactive seeds. Of course, for ten to twelve years, researchers have been playing with cryoprobe technology and freezing the prostate. There are indications for freezing the prostate, however, that this technique carries a lot of morbidity, such as incontinence and rectal fistula formation. The newer endoprobes have worked out the templates the same as putting in seeds. Theoretically, they could go ahead and freeze the prostate, then treat patients with external beam radiation.

There would probably be a better cure rate, and possibly less morbidity, than with seeds plus external beams. This technology is evolving, and there is a lot of competition among researchers to come up with innovative approaches.

With the current treatment options, I am thoroughly convinced there is nothing as good as surgery for the patient who is sixty-five or younger, especially if he is healthy and has curable prostate cancer. On the other hand, I'm very optimistic that the prognosis of patients with hormonal resistant prostate cancer (HRPC) will improve dramatically in the very near future.

Urologic Research

There are new medical research companies starting all the time, and many of them are concentrating on urologic problems. We have a new PSA test that can help us determine definitively if a patient has cancer or not. When you biopsy a PSA-positive patient three, four, or five times and they are still negative, then the question becomes, "When is enough, enough?"

I mentioned thermal therapy with its heating and cooling elements done in the doctor's office rather than in the hospital. It has all but replaced the TURPs we used to do for benign prostatic hyperplasia (BPH). I am not totally convinced that thermal therapy can replace a well-done TUR. The thermal method requires a patient wear a catheter for two weeks or more with frequent heavy doses of antibiotics. I'm from the old school, I guess.

There have been so many advances in my field of urology it is hard to cover them all in a short period of time. But advances have been steady and they have been dramatic. Take microsurgery, for example. It has so many uses in procedures such as renal transplantation and for men wanting to reverse vasectomies, just to name a couple. In the 1970s microsurgery had its beginning, and new applications for its use occur every year.

Organized Medicine

I think my earliest involvement in organized medicine came when a lot of talk began about the medical school in Reno going to four years (1977). Drs. David Johnson and Hoyt Miles got me involved, and I remember one of the first state medical association meetings I attended on the subject was in Las Vegas. The plane I was going to fly down in was past due for its annual inspection, so my wife, Pati, and I piled into the next one in line and had quite a ride. It seems on takeoff the cabin door was not properly secured and popped open over Walker Lake at about 14,500 feet. I put the plane, a Beach Debonair, into a stall in order to close it. Papers, maps, and lots of stuff, even the book she was reading, went flying out. As this was my first night flight to Las Vegas and all the maps were floating in Walker Lake, I contacted the airport and they flashed the proper runway lights for my landing. I'd say that was a good introduction to organized medicine.

When I was Nevada State Medical Association president, in 1992-1993, I thought doctors in the northern part of the state really ought to have better relations with our colleagues in the south. There was sort of an understanding that an on-going north-south rift was in play at any given time. Anyway, I set up meetings just to go down and find out what our differences were and why we were as far apart as we seemingly were. Nobody came to those meetings and it didn't take long to figure out I wouldn't be spending a lot of time doing that anymore. I guess when you're as reasonably unsophisticated and naïve as I was, ideas such as that can pop into your head.

We had high hopes for gaining a solution to the professional liability insurance problem in the 1993 legislative session, but in spite of having an effective coalition of concerned and involved associations and organizations, we did not gain the legislative tort reform package for which we had fought.

Looking Back

I look back on my career and wonder how it all went by so fast. I have enjoyed practicing quality medical care in Reno with my colleagues over the years, and I repeat that medical care in Reno was state-of-the-art when I got here in 1968. This quality has been maintained year after year after year. Medical technology has grown in leaps and bounds, the training of physicians has steadily improved, and our hospitals are among the best in the nation. I am very optimistic about the future of healthcare in this country.

What am I most proud of? That would have to be my children, but I have to credit my wife for bringing them up. The fact that they accepted the imposition the practice of medicine made on our family, without too much complaining, made the long hours and interruptions more tolerable. I don't see patients in the office anymore, but I do assist my partners two or three times each month at the hospitals. Time does pass quickly when you're busy doing nothing. My children have all been properly educated and have done remarkably well. My grandchildren are delightful, and my wife, Pati, keeps me forever young. I'm having the time of my life. I have enjoyed it all and am enjoying every minute of it right now.

Epilogue

Northern Nevada holds as much attraction today for physicians as when it was "being discovered" after the Second World War. In this book doctors related how they were attracted to this "edge of the desert" by friends in the profession and by northern Nevada's strategic location. Others were attracted by the magnificent outdoors, open spaces, mountain sports, desert, hunting and fishing, and there was a sense they came because of the growing economy, lack of traffic congestion, and a relaxed style of living. Once here, their perception that northern Nevada had an outstanding medical community was reinforced and, from testimonials contained herein, doctors held that belief throughout their careers.

Only one of nineteen physicians interviewed was a native to the Silver State. In fact, it was only later in the 1970s and '80s that increasing numbers of Nevada-born physicians began to stay and practice here. The University of Nevada School of Medicine led the way by graduating students who were born and raised in Nevada.

In the 1950s Nevada was a relatively inexpensive place to live. Gambling revenues were enough to keep personal taxes low and there was no sales tax. The statistics in the appendix give a snapshot of expenses in the forty-eight states during the 1950 decade.[1]

In the 1950s and '60s the practice of medicine was quite different from what it would become by the end of the century. Government was far less involved in medical affairs and far less intrusive in medical practice. Medicare and Medicaid came into being in the mid 1960s, but even then things were quite good for physicians. That may have been the end of the "Golden Age of Medicine" when doctors were able to practice unfettered medicine and were being paid a portion of their fees for medical care they formerly donated.

In the 1960s there were enough patients for Reno's doctors, and enough income to pay the bills. Patients were seldom, if ever, turned over to collection agencies. Few doctors interviewed for this book were from wealthy families and most worked their way through undergraduate school, medical school, and residency. One doctor reminisced about eating beans one night and corn the next night cooked on a hot plate in his room. Others reflected on their work in emergency rooms and doing construction work while in training.

Newly arrived northern Nevada doctors soon learned to prefer one particular hospital over the other. Some enjoyed practicing at the "County

187

Hospital," as Washoe Medical Center was called, because of its range of care and it had the only emergency room in northern Nevada. Others preferred St. Mary's Hospital, with its family oriented atmosphere. Still other doctors had no preference and used both. One noted that in the early days St. Mary's did not have an emergency room, and he could build his practice by taking patients who came in the ER at WMC.

Physicians' preference for Washoe Medical Center was due partly to its outstanding administrator, Carroll Ogren, who managed the hospital from 1964 to 1978. His support for purchasing new medical and technological equipment and building new facilities, combined with his trust in the medical staff, allowed the hospital to grow in reputation. Contributors to this book considered him a friend and recognized that his leadership kept the hospital on the cutting edge.

Hospitals were becoming monuments to expansion and competition. They became involved in developing a "seamless" healthcare system, or, as some pundits labeled them, a "Cradle to Grave" of healthcare providers. The hospitals were involved in regional systems of care and they proceeded to buy outlying hospitals and medical laboratories. They even entered the real estate business by buying and building magnificent office buildings to attract physicians. They became heavily involved in offering discounted rates to various health insurance plans to garner "market share." In short, hospitals were becoming economic giants with insatiable appetites.

Doctors who came to the area in the 1950s and 1960s were in for dramatic changes during the life of their practices. They would see Medicare and Medicaid become healthcare cost containment programs in addition to delivery systems. They would see federal government administrators finding ways to reduce reimbursement to doctors and hospitals.

"Managed Care" became the catch phrase for the new role insurers would play ostensibly to stabilize the dramatic rise in the costs of healthcare. Nevada held the dubious honor of having the highest healthcare cost in the nation for several decades and in the forefront of mechanisms for controlling these costs was the Health Maintenance Organization (HMO.) To enroll in an HMO plan, which was most times less expensive than conventional health insurance, patients only had to agree to give up their choice of family physicians, specialists, hospitals, and laboratory services. Furthermore, the "gatekeeper" specified what services, procedures, and medications were to be used. Too much to give up for costs containment? Perhaps, but even these containment measures did not stop the juggernaut of the increasing cost of healthcare. The medical profession also recognized the wisdom of containing costs. In the 1980s, the AMA urged the nation's physicians to freeze their fees for a year. Nevada doctors complied, but this measure had no effect on containing costs. The cost of new technology accelerated and new specialties with highly trained doctors doing high tech procedures evolved.

These new specialties are providing excellent coverage and services that were not formerly available. One medical specialist that has emerged in recent years is the hospitalist, whose entire role is treating hospital patients admitted by other physicians. Other specialists that have emerged in the last fifty years are neonatologists, perinatologists, gastroenterologists, radiologic oncologists, cytopathologists, and invasive radiologists, to name a few. Not all specialists have stood the test of time; for example, virtually all proctologists, have disappeared and were replaced by the gastroenterologist. Even specialties have changed; the general practitioner has become the family physician.

Some specialists had to give up areas of practice when new and highly trained doctors came to town. Some called this encroachment. Just to name a few, after cardiologists arrived doctors of internal medicine who had been taking care of patients with heart conditions began receiving fewer referrals from their colleagues. Radiologists who had been doing upper and lower GI barium imaging found fewer physicians ordering these tests after the gastroenterologists offered a more complete examination with an endoscope. Ophthalmologists gave up refraction and eyeglass business to optometrists, but it all seemed to workout.

The rising tide of medical specialization lifted the boats of many others involved in providing healthcare service. Those benefits were found in the rise of career opportunities for paramedical and technical assistants and a new classification of medical care providers arose to provide highly specialized care: Nurse Practitioners (NP), Advanced Practitioners of Nursing (APN), Certified Nurse Assistants (CAN), and radiological techs (CT, MRI, PET, mammogram, and sonogram techs). New non-technical careers were also formed within the managed care industry, such as prior authorization techs, provider relations representatives, length-of-stay specialists, staff who determined credentials, and physician's office staff skilled in insurance coding and insurance reimbursement. Out of these advances a place for highly compensated medical administrators developed.

The mini-biographies of physicians in this book clearly show that these well-trained specialists brought state-of-the-art surgical techniques and medical technology with them to Nevada. Throughout their careers they kept their skills current by attending education courses, seminars, and training sessions to provide high quality medical care.

There were, of course, some doctors who came to the Reno-Sparks area who left for unknown reasons. A few physicians went off to gain extra training and did not return, and some left to change specialties. Some retired and moved elsewhere, but the overwhelming majority of doctors who located in northern Nevada stayed the course and raised their families here. Each doctor quoted in this book relates satisfaction at making that choice to come to this community. Each has made substantial contributions not only to medicine and the advancement of quality healthcare, but also to the northern Nevada civic community as well.

APPENDIX

Cost of Living in the United States

Item	1950	2003	Increase
Average annual income	$4,500	$25,000	5.6X
Hourly minimum wage	75¢	$5.75	7.7X
Average home purchase	$17,000	$150,000	8.3X
Medium priced auto	$1,850	$13,000	7.0X
Gallon of gasoline	27¢	$1.70	6.3X
Loaf of bread	16¢	$1.75	10.9X
Postage stamp	3¢	37¢	12.3X
Gallon of milk	96¢	$2.00	2.1X

Medical Costs in Reno

General practice visit	$3	$100	33.3X
House call	$5	—	—
Specialists visit	$5	$200	40.0X
Hospital stay per day	$25	$1,200	48.0X
*Chest x-ray	$10	$96	9.6X
*Complete blood count	$5	$57	11.4X
*Urinalysis	$3	$34	11.3X
*EKG	$10	$75	7.5X
*Paps smear	$5	$40	8.0X

* Designates outpatient charges. Inpatient charges at local hospitals are considerably higher reflecting added overhead charges. These comparisons are only a rough guide to present day charges because various private, state government, and federal government programs have negotiated different charges.

Selected Bibliography

Printed Sources

Ackerknecht, Erwin H., *A short History of Medicine* (Balto.: Johns Hopkins Univ. Press, 1982).

Moss, Arthur et al, "Prophylactic Implantation of a Defibrillator in Patients with Myocardial Infarction and Reduced Ejection Fraction" NEJM, March 21, 2002, Vol. 346, No. 12, pp.877-83.

Naples magazine (Naples, Florida 2003).

Nevada State Medical Society minutes, 1915. (Unpublished, in the Univ. of Nevada School of Medicine history of medicine archives).

Pugh, Richard, *Serving Medicine: The Politics of Medicine and Nevada State Medical Association* (Reno: Greasewood Press, 2002).

Sohn, Anton, *A Saw, Pocket Instruments, and Two Ounces of Whiskey: Frontier Military Medicine in the Great Basin* (Spokane: Arthur Clark, 1998,).

Sohn, Anton and Carroll W. Ogren, *People Make the Hospital: The History of Washoe Medical Center* (Reno: Greasewood Press, 1998).

Interviews

Dr. Ronald Cudek, January 8, 2003
Dr. Theodore Berndt, November 4, 2002
Dr. Rodney Sage, July 2002
Dr. John M. Davis, June 7, 2001
Dr. Frank E. Roberts, May 8, 2001
Dr. Adolph Rosenauer, August 7, 2002
Dr. Ronald Avery, September 24, 2002
Dr. George Magee, November 19, 2001
Dr. Jack Talsma, June 25, 2002
Dr. Charles McCuskey, January 20, 2003
Dr. Bud West, January 23, 2003
Dr. Owen Bolstad, 2001
Dr. Anton Sohn, 2001
Dr. Francine Mannix, January 24, 2003
Dr. John Iliescu, October 31, 2001
Dr. John Chappel, July 2, 2003.
Dr. Frederick Boyden. November 26, 2002
Dr. Wes Hall, January 7, 2003
Dr. Joseph Reikemeyer, June 27, 2002

Index

Nitz, Gordon
  Reno urologist, 179
north-south rift, 186

O

O'Brien, William, 86, 126
  Reno anesth., 12
O'Callaghan, Michael
  Governor, 5
Ogren, Carroll, 47, 49, 50, 137,
  157, 168, 179, 188
  WMC admin., 20
Oppleman, Daniel
  UNSOM, 147
optometrists, 77
oral cancer, 160
orthopedic
  trauma, 89
Osmundson, Neil
  Bolstad's friend, 109
Ossman, Dr.
  Reinemeyer's friend, 177
osteoarthritis, 91
osteopaths, 93
overweight patients, 174

P

pain management, 14
Palmer, John, 126
  Reno peds., 47
Pap smear, 119
Paracelsus, 2
Parsons, Lawrence
  early Reno path., 111, 119
Pasutti, William, 126
  Reno peds., 47
path. dept.
  overthrow at WMC, 175

Pauly, Ira
  Reno psychiatrist, 182
  UNSOM psychiatrist, 152
Pemberton, Penelope
  Reno peds., 129
Peterson, Lowell
  Reno surg., 33
Phalen, J. Stephen
  Reno internist, 22, 33
Phy. Aid Committee, 163
physiatrists, 93
Plato, 3
pneumonia, 171
Pomeranz, Gary
  Reno assoc., 77
Pringle, Maida
  WMC nurse and admin., 49
Pritchard, Janice
  Reno Med. Plaza, 14
Professional Standards Review
  Organizations, 170
prostate cancer, 161, 181
prostate specific antigen, 184
psoriasis, 34
psychiatric drugs, 151
Pugh, Charlotte
  Rick Pugh's wife, 79
Pugh, Rick
  NSMA exec., 79

Q

Quaglieri, Charles
  Reno neurologist, 22
Quinn, Walter
  Reno physician, 90

R

radial keratotomy, 81
Rammelcamp, Charles
  Davis' teacher, 38

LIBRARY OF CONGRESS CATALOGING-IN-PUBLICATION DATA

Pugh, Richard G. 1938-
The cutting edge : reflections and memories by doctors on medical
advances in Reno/
Richard G. Pugh.

p. cm. – (The golden age of medicine in Nevada series ; 4)
Includes bibliographical references and index.
ISBN 0-9710267-0-X

1) Pugh, Richard G., 1938- 2. Physicians—Nevada—Reno—Biography. 3.
Medicine—Nevada—Reno—History. I. Title. II. Series.

R 277. P84 2003
610'.92'279355—dc21